THE **REVOLUTIONARY** KETAMINE

The Safe Drug That Effectively Treats Depression and Prevents Suicide

JOHNATHAN EDWARDS, MD
FOREWORD BY GAVIN DE BECKER

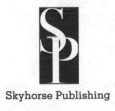

Skyhorse Publishing

Skyhorse Publishing books may be purchased in bulk at special discounts for sales promotion, corporate gifts, fund-raising, or educational purposes. Special editions can also be created to specifications. For details, contact the Special Sales Department, Skyhorse Publishing, 307 West 36th Street, 11th Floor, New York, NY 10018 or info@skyhorsepublishing.com.

Skyhorse® and Skyhorse Publishing® are registered trademarks of Skyhorse Publishing, Inc.®, a Delaware corporation.

Visit our website at www.skyhorsepublishing.com.

10 9 8 7 6 5 4 3 2 1

Library of Congress Cataloging-in-Publication Data is available on file.

Cover design by Kai Texel
Cover illustrations courtesy of Getty Images

Print ISBN: 978-1-5107-7771-2
Ebook ISBN: 978-1-5107-7795-8

Printed in the United States of America

To my parents and teachers, Bill and Susan Edwards, who provided me with everything possible. To the few high school and college teachers who were able to see past my impatience, and my coaches in all my sports who nurtured my motivations. To Gavin de Becker, who encouraged me after our discussion about ketamine. He truly cares about human beings and the cost of suicide to society.

To Dr. Sam Zand, who has helped countless patients in his psychiatry clinic and also reviewed the manuscript. Godspeed Ronn Bailey, for his invaluable support throughout the years. To Derek Du Chesne, Dana Gentry, Louie Amelburu, Sheldon Jacobs, Tom Insel, Dave Feifel, Joel Friedman, and everyone else to whom I owe my sincere gratitude.

And to my Uncle James Lawrence whose motivation, courage, and honor helped me, until his addiction finally took him—and his pain—away.

Even if this book saves a single life, it's worth all our effort.

Contents

Preface

Suicide. The word suicide is captivating. When I was only seven years old, my grandfather, recently diagnosed with chronic obstructive pulmonary disease (COPD) and given oxygen to live on, placed a shotgun to his chest and took his life. Just like that, he was gone through a single decision. At that age, I could not process what was going on and why someone would want to take their own life. My father explained that my grandfather was a Native American (he was born on a reservation), and he believed that it was better to take his own life than to exist unnaturally. Certainly, too much for a seven-year-old to process. I have thought about my grandfather's suicide just about every day since. I witnessed how the ordeal affected my father and even more my grandmother.

Later in my medical training, I discovered that tens of millions of others had been touched by suicide and the mental health crisis. Finally, when I was in private practice in Las Vegas, Nevada, I had five physician colleagues whose sons and daughters had all committed suicide before the age of eighteen. This struck me profoundly, and I have been a suicide prevention advocate ever since.

When most people think about suicide, they don't imagine a young child taking their own life. Suicide is the stuff of other people's nightmares. A mother losing her child to suicide is horrific, and the reality of that grief is insurmountable. No amount of therapy can make sense of what just happened or assuage the unimaginable pain. Time stops. The event continually replays in your head, leaving you wondering what you could have done differently. Getting support of any kind is a first step. A mental health provider can offer therapy, medications, and support groups. Most never see it coming. The subtle signs of mental illness often become apparent only after the fact. These signs are even more challenging to see in a young child.

In 2020, eighteen students committed suicide in Las Vegas, more than one hundred adolescents jumped from the Golden Gate Bridge in San Francisco, 228 US police officers committed suicide, and Hayden Hunstable took his own life just four days before his thirteenth birthday. Then there is the isolated case of Drew Robinson, a major league baseball player who thankfully survived his suicide attempt.

The COVID lockdowns were gasoline to the fire that is the existing mental-health crisis. More adults and adolescents are depressed than ever. While suicides during the lockdowns did not increase as many thought they would, the resulting increase in mental illness is undeniable. Worldwide, about 1 million people go through with the act and ultimately die each year.

Suicidal ideation is truly a hijacking of our brains, telling us to end our lives prematurely. What if there were a way to radically alter this hijacking device and grant the person in pain time to work things out, perhaps even losing the desire to take their own life? Ketamine is the one drug we have available to us today that can stop suicide in its tracks. Most have never heard of ketamine and, even among those who have, few know it could be used for seriously impacting the rate of suicide. Ketamine is not the final answer in ending suicide, but it is one very significant tool we have that can change the course of a never-ending scourge.

After reading this book, you will fully understand what suicide is, possible steps for prevention, and its devastating cost to our society. To those who say more studies are needed to know if ketamine helps with suicide and depression, I offer you this admonition: if you are that person suffering from depression and suicide, the risk versus reward is clearly in favor of using ketamine now. This book brings together many aspects of the mental-health crisis, suicidality, and how ketamine can help. Throughout this book, you will encounter many stories about suicide, mental health, addiction, and how ketamine changed the course. Ketamine has been safely used for over seventy years. There are scores of publications about ketamine; about 6,500 papers exist in the Medline/PubMed database. Today, these findings and data may be at their most important as the world we live in continues to lose its bet to suicide.

This book is dedicated to the invisible lives lost by suicide.

Foreword

Every suicide ends one life—but rolls a grenade into the lives of many others. I saw that happen to my family when my mother ended her life, and like all family members who experience suicide, I've felt it every day since, despite fifty years having passed. Suicide is a tragedy that is usually preceded by lots of pain, the ending being only the most dramatic moment in lives with plenty of drama.

In recent years, we all got a closer glimpse into suffering. The use of mass lockdowns had many consequences unrelated to a virus: the social order upended, bringing crime spikes, economic destruction, job loss, poverty, anxiety, isolation from loved ones and friends, alienation, drug and alcohol abuse, depression, and hopelessness. Those last items—isolation, alienation, depression, and hopelessness—are the four horsemen of the personal apocalypse, and they are stampeding through our society today.

During a low point, when people needed connection, companionship, and community, many governments ordered that we stay at home, isolate, separate, distance, cover our faces, and touch no one. When an elderly husband went to the hospital in 2020 and 2021, he went alone. His spouse watched him taken out of their home and never saw him again. He died alone, and she mourned alone. More than 1.5 million Americans died in hospitals in 2020 from all causes (not just COVID-19), and almost all died alone.

There is another group of people who usually die alone: those who suffer so much that they want to end their lives, which tens of thousands of Americans do every year. And despite this never-ending epidemic of suicide, few people are aware that a safe treatment exists, a treatment that often brings immediate improvement and immediate reduction in suicidality: ketamine.

Ketamine has been FDA-approved for decades; it's the anesthesia of choice for children because of its excellent safety profile. We know the dose for the treatment of depression is safe because it is one-tenth the dose that's been used millions of times for anesthesiology.

As long ago as 2010, the *New York Times* reported:

It has been known for several years that small doses of ketamine can relieve major depression.

Said Maggie, 53, "I woke up the next morning, and I didn't take an antidepressant for the first time in 20 years."

"I look at the cost of not using ketamine—for me, it was certain death," said Dennis Hartman, 48, a businessman from Seattle.

He said that after a lifetime of severe depression, he had already chosen a suicide date when he entered a clinical trial of ketamine at the National Institutes of Health two years ago. His depression lifted, and since then, he has gone to a clinic in New York every two months or so for infusions.

In a 2012 study published in the journal *Science*, the authors called ketamine, "the most important discovery in half a century."[1]

Since depression is among the world's leading causes of death, and since there is an effective drug that's available, safe, and inexpensive, how could it be that almost no doctors know any of what you've just read here?

That's precisely why one medical pioneer, Dr. Johnathan Edwards, dug deep into the research, conducted his own studies, added his profound compassion, and ultimately wrote this book. Rather than merely studying the sad statistics, Dr. Edwards committed to helping those who need never become statistics at all.

Thank you, Johnathan, for your work that improves and saves lives and for writing this book that will help others do the same.

—Gavin de Becker, bestselling author of *The Gift of Fear*

CHAPTER ONE

Suicide. Why Ketamine?

"All it takes is one small change on the earth to make a world of difference."

—*Anonymous*

Thomas Insel, MD, the leading voice of the psychiatric establishment in America and former director of the Mental National Institutes of Health, explains:

> Modern medicine has been successful at bending the curve, or decreasing deaths, in almost every disease known to man—cardiovascular disease, cancer, diabetes, malaria, and others. But suicides have never decreased in over thirty years, despite increasing awareness and numerous medications for suicide and depression.[1]

More people die from suicide than in all wars and homicides combined. It affects all individuals, every nation, race, culture, religion, and gender. According to the World Health Organization (WHO), the global suicide rate for nearly all ages has been increasing for thirty years.[2] The rate rises and falls with pandemics and financial crises. In the US, it has been increasing over the last twenty years, and today, suicide is the third leading cause of death in young adults 15–24, behind injuries and homicide; in adults 35–44, it is the fourth leading cause of death, behind injuries, cardiac death, and cancer.[3, 4] Suicide normally hovers among the top ten leading causes of death in the US.[5]

We define suicide as death caused by self-directed injurious behavior with the intent to die. Perhaps strangely, humans are the only animals that ever commit suicide;[6] nearly a million people do so annually. Suicidal ideation refers to thinking about, considering, or planning on suicide; about 1.2 million Americans have these ideations each year. According to the US Data, firearms are the most common method of suicide, followed by suffocation and poisoning.[7] Suicide is a public health crisis that nobody is discussing. Yet, when asked, nearly 100 percent of adults believe suicide is preventable.

Globally, the WHO estimates that 800,000 people die from suicide yearly. Still, the actual number is likely higher, representing a global suicide rate of one death every forty seconds, and estimates project that this rate will shift to one every twenty seconds. Surprisingly, the highest suicide rates occur in Lithuania, Guyana, and South Korea.[8] In the US, suicide is a grave problem, taking the lives of over 46,000 people in 2020 and over 48,000 in 2021, comparable to the number of deaths from automobile accidents.[9] Surprisingly, there are twice as many suicides as homicides in the United States, and more Americans have died from suicide than during all wars since Vietnam.[10, 11] Even worse, if we were to erect a memorial for all who have died from suicide, it would be miles long.

Undeniably, the lockdowns during the pandemic increased mental health disorders, which contributed to many of these suicides and contributed to the number of drug-induced overdose deaths. Have we adequately considered the long-term unintended consequences? We are not discussing medical complications like respiratory, cardiac, or kidney diseases—instead, the deluge of mental health problems like depression, suicide, and drug overdoses. Of course, depression, suicide, and drug overdoses were problems long before the recent pandemic. Lockdowns and war have fueled a litany of tragedies in addition to suicides: heightened crime, starvation, financial ruin, and much more.[12, 13] Even in those pockets where actual suicides have not increased, depression, drug abuse, and suicidal ideation have—dramatically. At a low point in our society, when people needed connection, companionship, and community, many government plans called for people to stay at home and isolate.[14] Millions lost their jobs while gun, drug, and alcohol sales continue to rise.[15, 16, 17]

UNICEF predicted millions of people would die of hunger and postponed medical treatments, a potential outcome that, unfortunately, drew less notice.[18] We can now see some of those consequences in the uptick in excess mortality and the increase of malaria in poorer nations.[19] In addition, many traditional mental-health resources were removed as if rubbing salt in the wound. Death from suicide is an inconvenient truth, and the mental-health consequences will persist long afterward.[20]

Despite what you've just read, it is rare to hear about suicides, even though one happens about every twelve minutes according to the American Foundation for Suicide Prevention. Adolescent and adult mental illnesses have skyrocketed, and the tsunami of post-traumatic stress, depression, and suicides will follow. In 2020, eighteen Las Vegas students, all children, took their lives; more police officers died by suicide using their firearms than in the line of duty; four police officers who responded to the January 6 attack on the US Capitol died of suicide. More firefighters die of suicide than in burning buildings. Frontline healthcare professionals have a much higher risk of having depression, anxiety, insomnia, and distress. Rarely do these suicides draw adequate media attention.

Why does one decide to die by suicide? No one can fully answer that question, but biological, psychological, social, spiritual, and environmental factors influence depression and suicide. For about 130 Americans per day, it's the last worldly decision they'll ever make. Recent unfortunate suicides include beloved NFL superstar Junior Seau, actor Robin Williams, television personality Anthony Bourdain, and fashion designer Kate Spade. What contributing factors need to coalesce to bring someone to this life-ending decision? To most, the thought is terrifying and comprehension impossible. For others, attempting suicide is the only answer remaining to squelch their anguish.

Fear, self-isolation, and social distancing exacerbate the detrimental effects on those with and without mental illness. Our life experiences, traumas, emotional conflicts, and stories sculpt our psyche. A dark, self-loathing psychological perspective is required to bring a person to extreme measures. If someone is ready for suicide, their thought processes have hit a cul-de-sac, which is sardonically French for "dead-end." Suicide is subtle, and the decision to take one's own life is often impulsive. Rigid thought patterns inhibit people with suicidal ideations from reaching out for help. Our daily environment, habits, stressors, and relationships are strong influences. Consider what social distancing does to someone already practicing isolative and self-deprecating behaviors. The spiritual elements of life include questions like, what's the point of all this? Why are we here? What happens after we pass? There are no correct answers here. Those who have misaligned their spiritual truths find it harder to discover a sense of peace and empowerment. Life lacks significance for those without purpose, appreciation, or a sense of enjoyment. When a loved one takes their own life, they leave many unanswered questions; constant thoughts of "what" and "why" permeate the minds of those left behind.

Suicidality is extraordinarily difficult to assess, and the field of psychiatry is left to treat an illness not fully understood. Treating suicide and depression is complex, and psychiatrists and other mental health professionals will attest that few medications can effectively treat suicide or treatment-resistant depression. Medicines for depression and suicide take weeks to have an effect; faster-acting antidepressant medications are needed to treat and prevent suicides.[21]

What if there was a way to remove the hijacking device leading to suicidal ideations and grant time to work things out? We have a little-known medication available today that can stop suicide in its tracks, and it's called ketamine. Most people have never heard of ketamine, and you might well be wondering how ketamine can be a game-changer for treating suicidal ideation, PTSD, addiction, and depression. Few are familiar with this decades-old anesthetic and party drug.[22] Ketamine can rapidly stop suicidal ideation and buy precious time to seek help and might save your loved one's or even your life. Ketamine is a legal and well-studied path to treat certain mental disorders, and four decades of research have transformed ketamine from an anesthetic to a routine outpatient treatment for mental disorders.[23, 24, 25]

The military uses ketamine to help war veterans recover from PTSD.[26] Additionally, intensive care unit specialists are using ketamine to treat the out-of-control inflammation that kills many afflicted with COVID-19.

Ketamine therapy is going mainstream with celebrities. Catherine Oxenberg, perhaps best known for her long-time role on the 1980s prime-time show *Dynasty*, says ketamine helped her overcome PTSD and chronic pain. Catherine is the daughter of Princess Elizabeth of Yugoslavia and Howard Oxenberg. Introduced to acting at an early age, she trained with the likes of Richard Burton (married to Elizabeth Taylor). The Oxenberg family experienced a rift when Catherine's daughter, India Oxenberg, became heavily involved with the secretive cult NXIVM.[27] After years of struggle, she succeeded in removing her daughter from the cult and was instrumental in taking the entire cult down, and the founder, Keith Ranier, was sent to prison for 120 years. Her book, *Captive: A Mother's Crusade to Save Her Daughter from a Terrifying Cult*, recounts the harrowing experience of extricating her daughter from the cult.

Once India was safely home from the cult, trauma struck again as the Oxenbergs lost their Malibu, California, home in the Woolsey fire of 2018. From these traumatic experiences, Catherine and India both experienced PTSD; ultimately, Catherine's body shut down after years of suffering from fibromyalgia and chronic pain syndrome. Catherine attempted every modality to cure her chronic pain and PTSD: medications, cognitive behavioral therapy (CBT), counseling, pausing her acting career, physical therapy, and more.

In the act of desperation, Catherine tried ketamine through the advice of friends. She went to a northern California clinic and received a ketamine infusion which gave her the first moment of hope that recovery was possible. She remarks that going through a ketamine psychedelic experience made the most significant change for her, helping to overcome PTSD and chronic pain issues. Likewise, India underwent ketamine treatments and was able to stabilize her PTSD.

Catherine and India are uniquely positioned to help those women who have suffered sexual trauma and now devote their lives to helping individuals and families recover from the devastating effects of unresolved trauma. Catherine also provided therapy to many defectors from the NXIVM cult, most of whom were victims of trafficking and have had suicidal ideations and attempted suicide due to their trauma. Today, they are strong advocates of ketamine therapy, and through the Catherine Oxenberg Foundation, they provide immersive programs for survivors of sexual assault and PTSD using psychedelic-assisted therapy.

People in suicidal crises require complex and unique care. Many run away from seeking help, fearing the system will institutionalize them against their will. Over 50 percent of all those who attempt suicide have no history of a mental health disorder.[28] As in a thick fog, people with suicidal ideation cannot see reality clearly, making it challenging to help them. Suicide risk and depression are increased because of the stigma toward individuals with mental illness and their families. The effects are worse in poor socioeconomic areas since inadequate welfare also compounds economic adversity.

Unfortunately, the modern medical system is ill-equipped to deal with mental health crises, namely suicide, satisfactorily. Our first response is to give medication and ignore the role of emotions or address the person's history of psychological trauma. Western medicine looks at mental illness solely as a biological problem when, in fact, it is highly complex.

Mental health is an embodiment of the mind, body, and spirit. The word "holistic" is characterized by the belief that the parts of something are interconnected and can be explained only by reference to the whole. In medicine, holistic care is the appropriate treatment of the whole person—the mind, body, and spirit—rather than just the symptoms of an illness. Pharmaceutical treatments do not target the root causes of diseases; instead, we advocate taking long-term medicines for disorders that seldom improve. The current medical paradigm commits an error when trying to isolate something and treat just that one thing.

A well-known addiction expert, Dr. Gabor Maté, eloquently states that mental illness is the body's expression of experiences, beliefs, and lifelong patterns of relations to self and the world.[29] The word healing comes from an old-English term that means "wholeness," and when we become whole, we can reconnect with ourselves and elevate our consciousness. Psychedelics like ketamine and synthetic and plant medicines help us to achieve healing.

Predicting human behavior is complex; people who decide to take their life prematurely come from all walks of life—the wealthy, the working-class adults, and the poor. Suicides are frequently called "senseless," but there are many reasons people become depressed and take their own lives. When we are alone, afraid, and feel all hope is lost, fear hijacks our minds and controls our actions. Denial of the reality in front of us delivers a captivating and beguiling effect. Life's highest-stakes questions can be answered.[30] What could I have done to get my loved one help? What resources were available to redirect the path? How can I keep my loved ones safer? Neither privilege nor poverty can take the negative energies of the mental health crisis away or offer protection from suicide. We constantly watch the news reports of the bodies from murders and violence, but no one is monitoring or reporting those who die by suicide. Bringing these issues into the conversation will allow action to prevent our loved ones and fellow human beings from suffering from depression and suicide.

A psychedelic experience creates a profound opportunity to be your authentic self and can be tremendously healing, helping us realize things on a deeper level than our ordinary consciousness permits. Ketamine can create deep insights and openings to the psyche, helping us to reestablish connections and honest truths. By opening truths, we are offered possibilities to move ahead and explore why we hurt so badly. Whether it's an ayahuasca ceremony or a therapeutic ketamine session, these experiences retune the brain's emotional apparatus. That being said, psychedelics are not a panacea or the end-all. Contrary to many enthusiasts, neither plant-based nor synthetic psychedelic medicines will transform healthcare or human consciousness by themselves.

Hundreds of articles in news outlets have highlighted the benefits and growing interest in using ketamine and other psychedelics in treating mental illness.[31] As a result, they are becoming increasingly popular in mainstream medicine. Psychedelics are not intended to be taken daily to keep you in an altered state. Presently, psychedelic treatments are costly and time intensive and insurance does not generally pay for them, so they remain beyond most people's reach. We would be negligent to exclude and disregard their healing potential. Ideally, they help facilitate your access to a renewed connection with yourself and the world long after your experience.

Everyone needs to be aware of and knowledgeable about suicide in order to help an individual suffering from suicidal ideation. But despite the tragedies, disturbing statistics, and heartbreaking stories that have collectively gripped the world, we can draw from the lessons of these victims and look to a brighter future. Mental-health practitioners are employing everything, including telemedicine, to help people battle this threat.

****

Case Study: Derek Du Chesne
The Weight of Entrepreneurship: Success, Burn Out, Suicide,
& Self-Love and How Ketamine Saved My Life

The journey from idea to creation can always be challenging. When you dream of success, it all starts with an *idea*—the problem you will solve. These ideas can make us feel unstoppable, like a superhero, giving us euphoria, creativity, and rich emotions.

I went to Hollywood at 16, became a stuntman in the film *Transformers 2*, and then acted alongside Robert DeNiro, Dave Bautista, and Bruce Willis in feature films. A dream come true for a small-town Wisconsin kid. After acting, I then transitioned to running a non-psychoactive cannabis supply company. It's been quite an adventure.

My shift into business happened after witnessing my mother battling cancer, multiple sclerosis, and fibromyalgia, which led me to explore alternative medicines. Western medicine continued to fail her, overprescribing harmful pharmaceuticals to counteract the side effects of the others. A palliative care clinic started treating her with high CBD, helping her to wean off other medications, and this experience inspired me to start a new business called Healing Ventures.

I managed the business to the point that I had little time for sleep. Accounting, payroll, legal, HR, marketing, supply chain, your team, and family come first. There isn't enough time in the day to put a dent in the workload, much less for self-love. As entrepreneurs, we tend to prioritize our personal needs over mental wellness. Sixteen-plus hour workdays, sleeping at the office, new time zones every week, living in hotels, conferences, expos, meetings on meetings . . . keeping to a routine seems impossible. When we're determined to solve big problems, we neglect our own. Neglecting your needs could cost you everything in the long run. Don't be like me.

After the 2018 Farm Bill passed, every pharmaceutical, tobacco, cosmetics, food and beverage, wellness, and pet expo turned into the "CBD show." I thought I was living my dream, traveling 300+ days a year and visiting over forty countries. Growing up, I didn't have a passport, and this was my opportunity to see the world! Each day I was educating new audiences about the benefits of adding CBD to their products. The more new places I woke up, the harder it was to fall asleep. My doctor thought it would be a good idea to prescribe me Xanax for the weekly flights. When I couldn't focus, he prescribed Adderall (similar to every kid who acted up in school in the '90s). Quickly, Xanax lost its effect, and I couldn't stay asleep. Then my doctor said Trazodone would do the trick. It got to a point where I was taking Adderall along with Ambien. My productivity dropped, yet I would take another pill and power through. Eventually, it became overwhelming. The hustle-and-grind mentality of entrepreneurship led me to severe sleep deprivation and depression.

My company was on the brink of being acquired when I unexpectedly discovered that my partners were planning my severance package to avoid paying my share of the equity of the business that I helped build to $80 million in annual revenue and over 300 employees. A few weeks later, I discovered that the woman I thought was the love of my life wasn't faithful and blamed me for working too much. After nearly three years of living a dream come true, everything crumbled. I went from having life figured out to being suicidal. I built my identity entirely on business relationships; when those diminished, so did my light.

Months passed, and I was a shell of a human being. Barely eating or sleeping, not showering . . . I didn't even resemble the driven, happy, and loving person I had once been. Comprehending that level of loss, betrayal, shame, blame, guilt, and spinning in the "what-ifs" was devouring my soul. They were the darkest months of my life, and I wouldn't leave the house, sitting on my couch watching the sun rise and set while staring at the Xanax bottle next to the tequila. I couldn't help thinking the world would be better off without me. The only thing holding me together was how I couldn't do this to my mom. I was drowning, and everyone around me was breathing. I was devoid of connection to myself or the outside world. Nobody could understand me, and I couldn't understand them.

A friend of mine came over and told me that he was taking me someplace and that I needed help. It was a ketamine clinic. Initially, I was reluctant. My entire ethos was plant-based medicine, and I didn't need a "horse tranquilizer" to feel better. Not understanding or being educated on the benefits of ketamine therapy for depression, I didn't go with him. The next day, my friend came back while I was staring at the lethal cocktail of Xanax and tequila, and I thought, *What do I have to lose?*

After glimpsing the Harvard diploma, I felt more reassured at the ketamine clinic. After telling the doctor why I was there, he abruptly cut me off and asked if I had ever tried mushrooms or psychedelics. He reassured me I would be fine, brought me into another room, took my vitals, and inserted an intravenous line. There was zero treatment preparation. They gave me a sleep mask and headphones, and within a minute, I was on the most incredible journey. For the first time in months, the repetitive negative thoughts I was drowning in dissipated! It was like an immediate vacation from my brain, like I had just stepped off the hamster wheel for the first time since losing my sense of identity. The colors, the music, the detachment from my thoughts, and realizing that we are not our thoughts blew me away. I smiled and laughed at the fact that just a few minutes ago, I was contemplating taking my own life. That seemed silly, and it was an instant reminder of how beautiful life is—an immediate shift in perspective.

That first ketamine treatment was the single most profound moment in my life. How many other people's ambitions lead to burnout and then suicidal ideation? How many other people are struggling with similar things? How many others neglect to fill their cups with self-love and self-care? After my session, all I wanted to do was talk about it. How is it that I've spent years in alternative medicine and didn't know ketamine was an option to improve my mental wellness? Thankfully, ketamine therapy helped me achieve a neurological reset and reminded me of who I am—wiping away burnout and depression almost immediately. After ketamine, I said goodbye to my ego.[32]

The Road from a Wartime Anesthetic to a Party Drug to a Legitimate Medication for Treating Mental Illness

Alice laughed: "There's no use trying," she said, "one can't believe impossible things."

—Lewis Carroll, *Alice in Wonderland*

Ketamine's history is intriguing. It started as a research idea in the 1960s, then developed into a research drug, then an anesthetic; it was popularized in the Vietnam war, it became a party drug, and ultimately, it was recognized as something that could stop suicide.[1, 2, 3] In the late '90s, Yale University researchers gave ketamine to depressed patients in a small research study and, astonishingly, ketamine put their depression into remission. Later, they gave ketamine infusions to patients with major depression and suicidal ideation and again found it stopped suicidal ideations in many of the patients, certainly more than they expected. Today, hundreds of research studies demonstrate that ketamine is effective for mental illness: depression, suicide, addiction, PTSD, eating disorders, and neuropathic pain.

The 1960s

Anesthesiologists complained that the anesthetic phencyclidine was causing intense, prolonged delirium in patients following surgery, making it undesirable for human use. Parke-Davis (a subsidiary of Pfizer) directed efforts to synthesize a less potent form of phencyclidine. In 1962, chemists at Wayne State University synthesized a molecule called CI-581 and, shortly after, called it ketamine. Animal and human studies demonstrated that ketamine was remarkably safe, and in 1964, they tested it on twenty human volunteer prisoners and found the drug did not stop breathing or decrease blood pressure. This made it an ideal anesthetic. Still, it caused vivid hallucinations and dissociated people from reality, but not nearly as badly as phencyclidine. Ketamine became the perfect anesthetic for surgeries for both humans and animals.

The 1970s

Following the promising trials, the FDA approved ketamine for medical use in 1970. A highly effective, safe anesthetic, ketamine gained popularity during the Vietnam war for its use on the battlefield. Known as a "buddy drug," an injured soldier could be given ketamine to ease the pain until they could get to help. In the MASH units, surgeons could anesthetize patients without needing medical oxygen or blood pressure medications. Anesthesiologists started using ketamine to sedate children before surgery. These are reasons why ketamine is listed by the WHO as an essential medication and is the most used anesthetic in the world.

Throughout the 1970s, psychiatric and academic research on the effects of ketamine began. One of the earliest accounts of ketamine's use as a psychedelic was by a Mexican physician-psychotherapist named Salvador Roquet.[4] Roquet became world famous for his psychedelic treatments; hundreds of people in his clinics underwent traditional plant-based psychedelic rituals supplemented with ketamine treatments. However, he was a controversial figure in Mexico because of his questionable participation in the psychedelic interrogation of prisoners held by the Federal Police. Allegedly, he did not cooperate with the Mexican Federal Police, his clinics were shut down, and they imprisoned him for a time. Around 1978, the prominent physician, researcher, and mystic John Lilly self-administered ketamine to induce an altered state of consciousness. He summarized his experiences as "a peeping Tom at the keyhole of eternity." He wrote a book called *The Scientist: A Metaphysical Autobiography*.

The 1980s

Ketamine's use as a party drug increased in the 1980s, spreading across the US, Europe, and Asia. Around this time, powder and capsule forms of the drug appeared on the street. Partygoers used ketamine at raves. At sufficiently high doses, users experienced what is called the "K-hole" or the "multi-verse," which is a state of dissociation with visual and auditory hallucinations.

The 1990s

In hospitals, emergency room physicians, anesthesiologists, and veterinarians used ketamine a lot. But on the street, it was widely abused, taking on the names "Special K" and "Kiddy Smack," and ketamine's illicit use began to dominate the conversation around it. Even today, Asia still battles illicit ketamine use. In Russia, Vladimir Putin banned ketamine outright to fight its abuse. French actress and animal rights activist Bridget Bardot petitioned President Putin to allow ketamine for animals.[5] Putin removed the ban on veterinary medicine but still forbade its use in humans, which was unfortunate, considering that ketamine is an excellent anesthetic. In the late '90s, the DEA changed ketamine to a federally controlled substance to cease its illicit use. This did decrease the use of ketamine on the streets; however, other drugs like morphine, heroin, and cocaine became more prevalent among recreational drug users.

In 1998, researchers from the University of Cambridge successfully treated eating disorders like anorexia nervosa and bulimia with ketamine,[6] which gained international attention. This led to a series of important studies by psychiatrist and researcher Dr. John Krystal, who started experimenting with ketamine and its psychological properties and molecular mechanisms. The unanticipated finding was that ketamine also had antidepressant effects in patients.[7]

The 2000s

Nearly fifty years later, ketamine became a hot emerging topic in psychiatry. Studies from Yale University showed that ketamine produces a rapid suppression of suicidal ideation, which is unprecedented in psychiatry. Ketamine became a viable treatment for mental disorders, leading doctors to use ketamine off-label to treat mental disorders in ketamine clinics. In 2000, Yale University researchers such as Dr. John Krystal pioneered the use of ketamine for severe depression. Dr. Robert Berman showed that a single sub-anesthetic dose of ketamine improved the mood and depression scores of depressed and schizophrenic patients.[8] A compelling accumulation of data followed, showing a robust and relatively sustained antidepressant effect. They hypothesized ketamine could help in understanding the symptoms of schizophrenia because of its dissociative effects. Interestingly, research revealed that ketamine triggers an increase in glutamate, which prompts the brain to form new neural connections called neuroplasticity and makes the brain more adaptable and able to create new pathways, helping patients to reinforce positive thoughts and behaviors.

If ketamine is so good at treating depression and suicide, why didn't we know earlier? Well, it turns out that we did. Several physicians and researchers wrote about the antidepressant effects of ketamine early in the 1970s.[9, 10] In Edward Domino's article, "Taming the Ketamine Tiger," he wrote:

"Many years ago, when I was a clinical pharmacologist working part-time at the Lafayette Clinic, I ran the drug abuse screening laboratory. I was often referred patients by the attending psychiatrists. Several referrals dealt with phencyclidine and ketamine drug abuse, especially in the late 1970s and early 1980s. A number of these patients were mentally depressed and taking various antidepressants. I remember one young lady, in particular, who was a chronic phencyclidine and later ketamine abuser. She had serious bouts of mental depression. I asked her why she took these illicit drugs rather than her usual antidepressant medications. Her answer was, 'Oh, doctor, my antidepressants don't work as well.' She stated that ketamine and phencyclidine worked quickly and were much better antidepressants, but they didn't last as long, so she took them again and again."

Ketamine and Depression

The discovery of ketamine's antidepressant action has been described as the most significant advancement in the treatment of depression and suicide in this century. As the former director of the Mental National Institutes of Health (MNIH), Dr. Thomas Insel, explained, "there have been no new medications for depression in the last fifty years, and ketamine is the first to show a profound difference in treating depression and suicide." Given that even a single dose of ketamine may cause a rapid reversal of depression and suicidal thoughts, there has been a surging interest in using ketamine as a therapeutic agent for depression. Currently, the standard treatment for depression for the last fifty years has been some form of psychotherapy and antidepressant medications such as Prozac or Lexapro. Once all medication and therapy options are exhausted, patients can undergo electroconvulsive therapy (ECT) and transcranial magnetic stimulation (TMS), which we will discuss in a later chapter. Depression is a broadly stigmatized and misunderstood mental illness, and people who disclose their depression have difficulty getting jobs and maintaining relationships. Importantly, depression is not just one thing; it exists as a myriad of symptoms. According to the MNIH, 21 million Americans experience major depression, and one-third have treatment-resistant depression.[11]

Ketamine's path from anesthetic to antidepressant originated in the late 1990s with work by Drs. John Krystal and Robert Berman.[12] They published a groundbreaking proof-of-concept study of seven depressed patients who received relatively small doses of ketamine. What followed was extraordinary. The patients experienced a rapid, unmistakable reduction in depressive symptoms after twenty-four hours, and the effect lasted days after the treatment. Putting this into perspective, traditional antidepressant medications take weeks to show any effect and must be taken daily. In the meantime, these patients continue to suffer from depression and risk self-harm and suicidal ideations. The encouraging results of Dr. Berman's study have been since replicated in subsequent studies, showing that 70 percent of depressed patients responded to a single treatment of a sub-anesthetic dose of ketamine.[13]

The next breakthrough for ketamine was in a more complex form of depression called treatment-resistant depression (TRD). The differences between depression and TRD are important to understand. Imagine battling symptoms of sadness, sleep disturbance, low energy, and thoughts of death or suicide lasting two or more weeks—this is the definition of depression. Now picture being depressed and trying several medications and therapies, only to discover that none work. This is treatment-resistant depression. In 2005, physicians showed that a sub-anesthetic dose of ketamine combined with cognitive behavior therapy (CBT) improved the symptoms of TRD.[14, 15] Many of these patients were on several medications and underwent ECT for several years with no real improvement.[16] A group out of Australia published a pair of intriguing case reports about TRD.[17] One patient had an eighteen-month history of TRD that was unsuccessfully treated with ECT and anti-depression medications: Citalopram, Mirtazapine, and Venlafaxine. They gave her a series of ketamine infusions over five days. Her Beck Depression Inventory (BDI) improved from 36 to 11 in four days, and she remained well one year later on just Citalopram. The second patient had sixteen years of depression unsuccessfully treated with Fluoxetine, Nefazodone, Mirtazapine, Venlafaxine, Amisulpride, Lithium, and ECT. A series of ketamine infusions were administered over five days, and his BDI improved from 52 to 9 in four days. He relapsed twice, after two months and eight months, and underwent two further five-day series of successful ketamine infusions. At twelve months, he remained well on lithium.

In 2006, an extensive trial studying the effect of ketamine infusions on patients with TRD showed improvement in symptoms after a single treatment.[18] Then another two trials in 2009 showed positive benefits in TRD patients.[19, 20] Since then, hundreds of studies have documented the beneficial effects of ketamine on depression.

* * * *

Case Study: Ashley Clayton[21]

Ashley Clayton had undergone seventeen ECT treatments for her chronic major depression. Simple tasks became challenging. Ashley's depression wasn't getting better and it was only a matter of time before her illness might turn deadly. Ashley's childhood was scarred with severe trauma and suicide attempts. Despite her depression, she made it through high school and university and became a psychologist. In 2014, stressful events caused her depression to return and her mental health declined.

Even with therapy she experienced anhedonia (the inability to feel pleasure). Desperate, she researched ketamine and connected with Dr. Gerard Sanacora at Yale University, who enrolled her in a ketamine trial. Following the treatment, she went home and described "feeling dramatically different . . . a miracle." She regained her love for her husband, which she had lost because of her depression. However, approximately two weeks later, her depression returned. She contemplated suicide again. Apparently, she was unable to receive ketamine again because of financial and Yale University policies, and they again offered her ECT treatments. She began a series of seventeen ECT treatments, which ultimately did not cure her depression. Somehow, nearly one year since the first ketamine treatment, she was able to receive another, and her doctors convinced the hospital administrators to provide her ketamine treatments every two to three weeks, depending on her symptoms. Ashley states, "Ketamine not only saved my life but has restored me to the joys and pains of full living. I feel like there is air to breathe for the first time in my life."

* * * *

Ketamine and Suicide

Can we stop suicide? The answer is a resounding "yes." One of the most profound things ketamine can do is quell the desire to take one's own life. As mentioned in the first chapter, if you or a loved one is suicidal, consider ketamine now.

Medicine is limited in treating suicidal ideation. Typically, patients with suicidal ideation are admitted to the psychiatric ward in a hospital and given anxiolytics, sedatives, and tranquilizers. While antidepressants might lessen the risk of suicide, they typically take several weeks to work. Similarly, lithium and clozapine are effective anti-suicidal drugs but do not work in the short term; the same is true for psychotherapy. Moreover, suicide occurs at uncomfortably high rates in psychiatric units during admission and after discharge; this is why rapid suppression of suicidal ideation is vital.

One of the best pieces of evidence showing that ketamine infusions decrease suicidality is a 2022 study by Dr. Lori Calabrese. She enrolled 235 suicidal patients aged fourteen to eighty-four who received six ketamine infusions over two to three weeks.[22] Suicidal ideations were stopped in most patients, some in as little as four hours. She convincingly demonstrated the rapid, safe, short-term, and persistent benefits of ketamine, revolutionizing the outpatient treatment of suicidal ideation. No other medication or treatment for suicidal ideation has ever stopped suicidal thinking in four hours. In Dr. Calabrese's words, "ketamine does not just make the suicidal thoughts easier to bear, it erases them." A single ketamine infusion can whet your appetite for how life could be, which is why several infusions are required.

In an interview, the former director of the National Institute of Mental Health, Thomas Insel, MD, and author of *Healing: Our Path From Mental Illness to Mental Health*, said that he envisions ketamine will one day be the standard of care for suicidal ideation in emergency departments (ED). Currently, there are no validated approaches to suicidal patients in the ED except admitting them to the psychiatric ward for 24/7 observation. Yale University physicians studied fourteen patients who presented to the ED with suicidal ideation per their Montgomery-Asberg Depression Rating Scale (MADRS) scores.[23] The mean MADRS scores were 40 before the ketamine infusions, and the score afterward was 8 for all but one patient, meaning that their suicidal ideations were practically resolved. Even more, the reduction in suicidal ideation lasted for at least ten days after the infusion.

* * * *

Case Study: Olive

Olive is typical of many patients with severe depression and suicidal ideation history. By age fifteen, doctors diagnosed Olive with generalized anxiety disorder, panic disorder, PTSD, and bipolar disorder. She went through all the traditional approaches with psychiatrists and psychologists to treat her psychiatric conditions, such as cognitive-behavioral therapy, psychotherapy, counseling, meditation, mindfulness, and yoga. Taking several medications like Prozac, Celexa, Zoloft, Lexapro, Effexor, and many others with little effect, she often felt hopeless and spent much of her time alone, crying and sad. For her, depression was cancer for her soul and hell for her spirit. By age twenty-seven, she had fought the severity of her illness, but residual depression and irritability lingered.

As time continued, Olive's outlook darkened until she felt her life was not worth living. She decided that suicide was her only option. Unable to take her own life by conventional means, she planned to travel to the Netherlands for assisted suicide. She painted a picture of "Autumn Lake," which depicted her thoughts of what heaven would look like. She wanted her mother to envision her in this lake after she was gone.

A doctor suggested Olive try ketamine. However, Olive had already arranged her assisted suicide. On the day she was leaving for the Netherlands, Olive decided to try the ketamine treatments. Under the direction of Dr. Gerald Grass, she underwent multiple ketamine infusions and was no longer suicidal. After three ketamine infusions over three days, Olive's suicidal ideation and her depression and anxiety were gone.

After the ketamine treatments, she describes her depression as being replaced with joy, and anxiety with tranquility. She describes her brain as calm and her heart filled with happiness and love. Olive's renewed passion for life has given her a second chance. She describes moving forward with confidence, knowing that if her symptoms return, she can return to the ketamine treatments. In short, Olive got her life back thanks to ketamine.

Source: Gerald Grass Clinic, used with permission.[24]

* * * *

Treating Addiction with Ketamine

The treatment of alcohol addiction with ketamine showed a 40 percent reduction in relapse rate at twelve months, which is incredible compared to traditional twelve-step programs like Alcoholics Anonymous.[25] In 2022, psychologist Celia Morgan performed similar studies to treat alcohol addiction. Her group saw significant reductions in alcohol consumption and increases in abstinence in patients who received ketamine-assisted psychotherapy (KAP).[26] The therapy-only arm of the study also fared well, but adding ketamine made nearly a 10 percent difference in most cases. Ketamine has also been used for addiction therapy to other drugs like heroin and cocaine.

Ketamine and PTSD

The enormous problem of veterans and suicide is disheartening—over twenty veterans die by suicide every day; this number is probably closer to forty. Soldiers with post-traumatic stress disorder (PTSD) are at increased risk of depression and suicide. PTSD is a precise physiological and psychological response to traumatic events.[27] When false alarms, like certain noises, songs, or events, trigger a PTSD reaction, the body automatically perceives the stress and reacts. Few pharmacotherapies have demonstrated efficacy in the treatment of PTSD. One of the newer applications of ketamine is its treatment for PTSD in adults and children;[28] the same is being done with MDMA.

MDMA, also known as "Molly" or "Ecstasy," shows remarkable efficacy in treating severe PTSD. The results of phase 3 clinical trials published in *Nature* found that 67 percent of participants who took MDMA no longer met the diagnostic criteria for PTSD, which is an amazing outcome for this hard-to-treat condition (Mitchell).[29]

Researchers at Boston Children's Hospital conducted a study in 2019 in which they gave ketamine to military combat soldiers diagnosed with PTSD.[30] The patients underwent a series of six one-hour infusions to induce dissociation or a psychedelic response. The researchers predicted ketamine would give the veterans a life-changing, transforming experience. Most of the veterans reported a remarkable change, where they had reduced symptoms of PTSD and established a "reset" of their negative thoughts and behaviors.

* * * *

Case Study: Mike Donnelly

US military veteran Mike Donnelly openly discusses how ketamine treatments have helped him. Because of his combat experiences and suffering from PTSD while serving with the Army National Guard in Iraq, he found himself at the "end of his rope." He tried to find help via the internet and the VA hospital system. Failing conventional medical therapy because of the side effects, he began feeling hopelessness and an ever-increasing frustration with the VA medical system. He describes a situation familiar to many service members who have PTSD and have reached out to the VA medical system. Mike managed as best he could for years and found himself on the brink of suicide when he walked into a VA hospital in West Haven, Connecticut, and asked to see someone about his issues. He was given a toll-free number to call for suicide prevention, a "pat on the back," and told to come back in a month to see how the medications were working. From that point, he explains that he spent six months trying to find the correct medicines at the proper dosage with little relief and became profoundly depressed. Unable to function as a father, husband, or employee, he destroyed his close friendships and began contemplating suicide using his firearm. He dove into self-help books and religion and stumbled upon a video about ketamine treatment that claimed to help PTSD symptoms.

He found a physician named Dr. Ang in Connecticut, but unfortunately, the cost of the treatment was prohibitive because his insurance denied any coverage for ketamine treatments. From this point, he recalls barely being able to get out of bed, take a shower, and eat. He eventually sold a prized rifle to raise the money needed for the ketamine treatments, which he later described as a good decision. Mike went through the ketamine treatments and secured financial support through a foundation called the Ketamine Fund. Mike regained a better life with himself and his family, essentially saving his life. He even lost his job during the COVID-19 crisis and handled it well.

Source: The Ketamine Fund website and personal communication with Zappy Zapolin and Warren Gumpel, 2021.

* * * *

Ketamine and Chronic Neuropathic Pain

Chronic pain syndromes such as migraines, fibromyalgia, and neuropathic pain can be effectively relieved by ketamine and other psychedelics.[31] Millions of people have chronic pain and have little chance of a cure, and some even resort to killing themselves to relieve the burden of their chronic pain. Early studies showed better postoperative pain control in surgical patients who were given ketamine with a general anesthetic.[32] This is particularly important for the millions who suffer from unrelenting, insurmountable chronic pain, desperately trying to regain a semblance of everyday life—physically, emotionally, and socially. Ketamine and other psychedelics are most effective when used with a multi-disciplinary approach.

A multitude of findings across a handful of chronic pain conditions alludes to the possibility that psychedelics can ease chronic pain for significant periods of time. Most of these studies exist in the form of case reports and small studies. However, not everyone is convinced that ketamine helps chronic pain.[33] Despite this, many physicians are turning to ketamine to treat chronic pain because large trials will take years. The same phenomenon happened with ketamine and depression; once physicians realized that ketamine could rapidly treat mental illness, many used it before the research trials came out. Psychedelics, coupled with psychotherapy, will change the way we experience pain.

Author and podcaster Tim Ferriss is a big advocate of psychedelic therapy.[34] Ferriss recently underwent six ketamine treatments for TRD. During his podcast with Dr. John Krystal, he describes the ketamine treatments as effective for his depression. Unexpectedly, ketamine also helped his chronic back pain, and the relief lasted for months; for years, he had tried many modalities to relieve his chronic pain, apparently without success.

Some reasons psychedelics help chronic pain:

Central pain response—some psychedelics bind to the receptors responsible for pain;

Dampen inflammation—ketamine and other psychedelics can decrease the inflammatory cascade;

Neuroplasticity—increases the ability of the brain to change and strengthen pathways;

BDNF and mTOR—ketamine and psychedelics produce (upregulate) these proteins (we will discuss this later).

Dr. Krystal cites a close relation between anxiety, depression, and pain. He reasons that ketamine helps manage the emotional response we have to pain. Depression and anxiety cause us to focus on the pain and may blow the pain response out of proportion. It may not be that the pain is felt more intensely, but changing the way we perceive and feel our pain when we are anxious or depressed influences the overall picture. Another way to think about how ketamine affects chronic pain is that the brain lessens its impact on the painful memory, not allowing it to dominate the body.

* * * *

Case Study: Beth Seikel

Ketamine. The word alone brought fear, anxiety, and a "no thank you" whenever it came up as a treatment option for my complex regional pain syndrome (CRPS). When I looked into this medication years ago, I uncovered stories of patients traveling to Germany and Mexico to undergo a medically induced coma to reap the benefits of the anesthetic. As a long-standing ICU/ED nurse, that wasn't a direction I felt comfortable with, so I continued to resist.

My years of apprehension about ketamine, including the possibility of needing a med-port (a small medical gadget placed under the skin, allowing a catheter or IV to connect to a vein), coupled with the financial burden this treatment would place on my family, kept my avoidance going. I didn't want to deal with the uncertainty of my insurance carrier not covering the cost of infusions.

But after twelve years of living with CRPS, I developed burning pains on my tongue, and my heightened sense of things that shouldn't be painful (clinically known as allodynia) was spreading up to my upper body and face. It was enough! Increasing burning pain pushed me past my comfort zone. It was time to try ketamine.

With a medical background, I immersed myself in understanding "central sensitization," that is, the role that glial cells and NMDA receptor antagonists have on this chronic complex condition and how ketamine could be part of a plan toward relief. I reviewed educational presentations and publications from the Reflex Sympathetic Dystrophy Syndrome Association, where I now volunteer, and slowly began to feel more confident about this potential approach.

At first, I thought I could just try ketamine lozenges (also called troches) but soon realized they would not be enough to support the NMDA receptors activated by CRPS. These sublingual doses seem to help more with managing pain flares; ketamine infusions, administered via IV, were now needed. In my case of CRPS, the pain escalated in a continual pain loop as my brain and spinal cord became more sensitized. I knew I needed to face my fears and give ketamine a try.

So, in spring 2019, with the support of my incredible husband, I arranged with my CRPS pain specialist in Rhode Island a plan to administer the infusions at his clinic. My husband and I booked a nearby hotel room where we would spend our nights after the infusions. The infusions would last four hours each, over eight days. I learned in advance that common side effects are short-lived, temporary, and reversible; they can include a dreamlike state, colorful dreams, dizziness, headaches, and vomiting/nausea. Some individuals can experience extreme hallucinations or confusion.

Before receiving a ketamine infusion, patients are advised to have a cardiac workup and psych consult as medical clearance to rule out any underlying conditions before starting treatment. With my medical clearance, I was ready to begin my journey.

Knowing there are everyday items that provide much comfort in managing my CRPS, I brought along my soft blanket, neck roll, and dark sunglasses. Wearing my orange RSDSA hat and shirt, I started my eight-day "loading doses" of ketamine with a positive attitude.

For me, the hardest part of the infusion was the IV access, as my veins had become fragile, thin, and non-cooperative. Thankfully, the staff could use pediatric IV cannulas.

During the eight-day infusions, the medical team would increase the ketamine dose as tolerated. As a nurse, I paid close attention to the regimen. Before and after each infusion, I would receive an IV ondansetron (Zofran) dose to minimize and prevent nausea. In addition, I received IV midazolam (Versed) before infusion and every hour during the infusions to minimize hallucinations. The team also used magnesium (which supports NMDA receptors) combined with my infusion for two days and a vitamin C injection to help support my nervous and immune systems.

With my husband next to me, and practitioners from the advanced cardiac life support team monitoring my pulse, blood pressure, EKG, etc., I felt safe in the quiet, dim-lit room, which included darkening curtains and a comfortable temperature. I chose to lie down during the infusions, but also had the option of a reclining chair.

The nurses were incredibly supportive throughout, especially as my ketamine dose increased, which led to some hallucinations and vivid dreams that were sometimes unsettling. But with a gentle warm touch and calm demeanor, the nurses always reoriented me and reminded me I was perfectly safe. They also encouraged me to rest and relax as I repeated my personal mantra: "reset my NMDA receptors."

As the eight days went by and the dose of ketamine steadily increased, I felt a strange sensation of being disconnected from my body during the infusions. Some of my hallucinations felt like looking through a kaleidoscope and seeing different colors and shapes. As the colors changed, it felt as though I was part of a movie clip on a beautiful ride. I also had several internal conversations with myself. Whenever I opened my eyes, I knew where I was, but the dreamlike state of disconnection returned as soon as I closed my eyes again. However, the gentle touch of the nurses always reminded me of where I was. The best part: I had *no* pain! My limbs felt like weightless clouds, light, cool, and free. Imagine, after twelve years of CRPS torture, not feeling any pain? It was simply incredible.

A couple of times, I used the restroom during the infusions. Geez, talk about feeling disconnected. The nurses stopped the infusion and brought over a walker. At first, I thought, "I don't need that." But as soon as I put my feet on the floor, I was thrilled to have the support. With the nurse holding my back, I made it to the restroom like a clown walking in oversized shoes.

After each infusion, my husband helped me return to our hotel, where I rested with my blanket and enjoyed my daily craving for coffee, a blueberry muffin, and a jelly doughnut. I took 5 mg of Valium each evening to help me feel less off-kilter (I sometimes felt a rocking motion while sleeping). Rarely, I took an extra Zofran for nausea.

After the eight-day loading dose, I felt a 30 percent reduction in pain intensity. I could not deny that I truly felt different, even "better."

Two weeks later, I returned to the clinic for a two-day ketamine booster infusion using the same protocol, including a dose of magnesium in one of the infusion bags. After the booster, I can honestly report that I had a 50 percent reduction in pain intensity and could feel the "reset" of my central nervous system. I was less jumpy and less agitated as well. I never imagined this would be possible, but I am so proud of myself for taking that leap of faith. While ketamine is not a cure, it felt truly miraculous for me.

After my initial infusions, my doctor sent me for routine follow-up bloodwork to monitor liver function (some studies have correlated long-term use of ketamine with liver damage). Thankfully, the lab results were all good. So, my treatment could continue.

I have increased my vitamin C intake, taking it before and after blood work and in connection with IV infusions, to minimize further CRPS trauma (some research has shown a positive association between the vitamin and complex regional pain syndrome, and it has always seemed to help me). I also found it helpful to use over-the-counter lozenges and oral rinses to minimize dry mouth, another side effect of ketamine.

Now, several months after my first infusion, I go to the clinic every six to eight weeks for a one-day ketamine booster following the same protocol. Interestingly, after some follow-up boosters, I have not noticed as significant a change as I did after the first infusion. However, the overall quality of my life is far better. My flares tend to increase as I approach the end of a six- to eight-week mark, and I have been able to use prescribed ketamine troches during those times. I am curious how this will all play out over the cold winter months since I started my ketamine infusion journey in the warmth of spring.

Source: Practical Pain Management. CPRS and My Ketamine Infusion Journey. Feb 2020, https://patient.practicalpainmanagement.com/conditions/ crps-rsd/crps-ketamine-infusion-journey.

* * * *

Ketamine and Autism Spectrum Disorder

The autism spectrum, also called autism spectrum disorder (ASD), is an array of psychological conditions characterized by differences in social interactions and communication styles, as well as severely restricted interests and repetitive behavior. MIT researcher Stephanie Seneff predicts that half of all kids could be diagnosed with ASD by 2025. Nearly 50 percent of children with ASD have perpetual displays of repetitive behaviors and an intense focus or narrow or restricted interests with overlying anxiety disorder and depression. The journey from suicidal ideations to suicidal behaviors is a circuitous road for people with autistic children, and they have unique risk factors compared with the non-autistic population. As reported by the CDC, the rate of ASD has skyrocketed from 1 in 150 in 2000 to 1 in 44 in 2018. Even more, suicidality is underappreciated in children with ASD, who are twice as likely to report suicidal thoughts.[35] A 2014 *Lancet* study reported that 66 percent reported suicidal ideations.[36]

The culmination of these factors unfortunately results in the children being institutionalized. And consider that thousands of parents and caretakers must care for these children; over 75 percent of caretakers experience depression.

Psychedelics have been used in autism; however, little work has directly investigated the role of ketamine in improving quality of life for autistic individuals or enhancing their ability to more harmoniously engage in various social and intellectual contexts. About a dozen small studies conducted from the late 1950s to the 1970s tested psychedelic compounds—mainly LSD and psilocybin in autistic children and adolescents.[37] To understand whether and how psychedelic compounds could potentially be used to improve the lives of autistic individuals, researchers must carefully delineate the underlying biology.

Ketamine has the potential to help with the many challenges faced by autistic individuals. The drug has an excellent safety record and is regularly given to autistic children before surgery. One study gave intranasal ketamine to twenty-one patients with ASD and found no significant impact on clinical tests, but the ketamine was well tolerated.

One area where ketamine could help with autistic individuals is regulating N-Methyl-D-Aspartate (NMDA) receptors in the brain; it is well-known that autistic humans have NMDA receptor dysfunction, thus opening up the possibility for drugs like ketamine which affect the NMDA receptors. One such study along these lines found that ketamine restored thalamic prefrontal cortex (PFC) connectivity in a mouse model of ASD.[38]

Activity-dependent neuroprotective protein (ADNP) syndrome is a rare genetic cause of ASD. Ketamine was given to children with ADNP in a pilot study, producing positive results. This supports continuing the ketamine clinical development program in ADNP syndrome and identifies functional endpoints for such a program.[39]

A sixty-year-old male veterinarian diagnosed as autistic with major depressive disorder and suicidality benefited from ketamine. Like many autistic individuals, he had been treated with multiple psychotropic medications, was admitted to inpatient care several times, and had suicide attempts. He chronically suffered from decreased social functioning, repetitive behavior, sensory hypersensitivity, anxiety, low mood, anhedonia, lack of energy, and suicidality. Despite intensive treatment with therapy and medications, he remained challenged by his condition and environmental circumstances and could not return to work. After taking ketamine, he reported that his depressive and suicidal challenges had disappeared, and his autism-related complaints had diminished. This case—together with previous clinical research—suggests that ketamine is likely to be effective against depression and suicidality and that ketamine is potentially effective for mitigating challenges associated with being autistic.

Recent interest in treating children with ASD using ketamine and other psychedelics has increased. The mechanism of action of ketamine closely overlaps with the theory of ASD as an atypical neural correlate of synaptic communication and neuronal networks.[40] A small trial published in 2018 yielded promising results. Eight autistic adults with low support needs received three non-drug prep sessions, then they took the psychedelic MDMA, and four took a placebo. Then three more non-drug prep sessions were followed by a dose session and then finally with three more non-drug sessions. Those who had taken MDMA experienced a marked reduction in social anxiety, as measured by a clinician-administered social anxiety scale—a sustained effect lasting several months. Afterward, the four people who had received the placebo were offered—and accepted—the option to take MDMA.[41]

Individual differences in people's biological responses to psychedelics may also be revealing. McAlonan and her colleagues are working to enroll forty autistic people whose autistic behaviors and processing differences have no known genetic cause, plus thirty non-autistic people, to study how small doses of psilocybin affect brain circuitry and responses to sensory stimuli. She says that "looking closely at the underlying biology can begin to identify patterns in these drugs and that there will be a difference in response to psilocybin in autistic individuals versus non-autistic controls."

Many companies are actively exploring psychedelics for conditions that frequently co-occur in autistic individuals. Though psychedelics may not work for everyone, they may be a step forward and provide optimism where, for now, little exists.

Another case worth considering is that of Aaron Paul Orsini, an autistic author, educator, and researcher who was saved from anxiety, depression, and suicidality following the intentional use of psilocybin, LSD, MDMA, and ketamine in his late twenties. Orsini has written extensively about his experiences and ongoing research, publishing three books on the subject: *Autism on Acid* (2019), *Autistic Psychedelic* (2021), and *Introduction to Psychedelic Autism* (2022). He estimates that he has communicated with over 5,000 autistic individuals who have written or attended his AutisticPsychedelic. com peer support group. Over the course of ten years of work, Orsini has helped progress the field as a public advocate, an educator, and a research coauthor to the University of London, where he and his team have been investigating the benefits of psychedelic use in autistic populations.[42]

Psychedelics have inspired new hope for treating many conditions, as they seem to be unlike any treatments currently available. You might be wondering how ketamine and other psychedelics can treat these conditions. In short, psychedelic medications have long been used to treat mental diseases.

Their benefits can be broken down into four effects:

1. Psychedelics produce a safe environment through enhanced fear extinction, and they go to the root of the psychological trauma. Whether from childhood, war, or whatever, psychedelics subconsciously bring up repressed traumas and allow the person to work and confront them in a safe, nurturing environment.

2. Psychedelics provide an anti-addictive benefit. Ketamine treats addiction to alcohol, cocaine, and opioids, along with psychotherapy, which is KAP (ketamine-assisted psychotherapy).

3. Psychedelics belong to a class of compounds known as psychoplastogens, which promote structural and functional neuroplasticity in the brain, creating new neural pathways.[43]

4. Finally, psychedelics bring a spiritual connection or a reconnection. Many of these effects are present long after taking psychedelics, and science has difficulty explaining this phenomenon. A spiritual connection helps some feel like a higher power put them on this earth and that we are all connected. It helps us realize that grass, animals, and the ecosystem are alive. Acceptance begins with allowing things to be as they are, with nothing to do with complacency or resignation. Psychedelics help now, and things cannot be other than how they are—accepting the difficulty of the situation or decreasing the resistance to accepting the situation. Psychedelics help you feel like you have a place to belong again, which answers many societal issues.

Is Ketamine Recognized as a Psychedelic Medicine?

Is ketamine a psychedelic? This question comes up a lot, and the short answer is yes. Based on the hallmarks of psychedelic experiences and the neurobiological definitions of psychedelics, it is accurate to state that ketamine is a "psychedelic" medicine.

Though ketamine's origins are as a dissociative anesthetic, it has become the primary medicinal application of psychedelic medicine. With proper dosage, setting, and preparation, ketamine can be entirely and genuinely psychedelic, encompassing the entire psychedelic experience.

Ketamine's classification as a psychedelic is essentially a matter of semantics. Clinical, academic, bioethical, and commercial entities disagree on the formal definition of "psychedelic." Some argue that ketamine is not a "classical psychedelic," which refers to hallucinogenic compounds that operate primarily on the serotonergic 5-HTA2 brain receptors. This group includes psilocybin (found in psychedelic mushrooms) and lysergic acid diethylamide (LSD). In comparison, ketamine acts on the brain's glutamate systems and NMDA receptors. Those who support ketamine's classification as a psychedelic cite its similarities to classical psychedelics' neurobiological (physical) and phenomenological (mental) characteristics. They also point to the similarity in patient outcomes through various psychedelic therapy modalities in clinical research, despite a difference in neurological mechanisms of action. Notably, Maltbie et al. used fMRI blood-oxygenation-level dependent signal (BOLD) response to show that glutaminergic signaling is not the only pathway involved in the BOLD response to ketamine and that 5-HT2A and dopamine are involved. Because 5-HT2A receptors in the PFC project to the ventral area, it holds that 5-HT2A receptors are well positioned anatomically to modulate the psychomimetic effects of ketamine.[44]

Ketamine is not alone in this discussion. The compound 3,4-methylenedioxymethamphetamine (MDMA) is another non-classical psychedelic with research-backed medicinal applications and FDA approval-tracking. MDMA has also been shown to lead to positive mental health outcomes, especially in patients with post-traumatic stress disorder (PTSD).

The recognition of ketamine as a psychedelic is larger than semantics: It is about increasing access to psychedelic therapy and improving mental health outcomes for patients. According to the US Substance Abuse and Mental Health Administration (SAMHA), 21 percent of US adults experienced mental illness in 2020, representing one in five adults or approximately 53 million individuals.

Psychedelic medicine research shows positive results for an increasing number of mental health conditions and their symptoms, such as:

- Mood disorders (depression, major depressive disorder, bipolar disorder)

- Anxiety disorders (generalized anxiety disorder, social anxiety disorder)
- Trauma disorders (PTSD)
- Substance use disorders (alcohol use disorder, substance use disorder)
- Suicidal ideation

"We know through research that all psychedelic compounds exhibit different felt experiences and neurobiological effects, even classical psychedelics within their category," Dr. Leonardo Vando, Mindbloom's medical director, says. "What is most important are the tremendous outcomes psychedelic medicines like ketamine, and FDA approval-tracked compounds like MDMA and psilocybin, are providing to clients living daily with mental health challenges."

While "psychedelic" remains an umbrella term, with most agreement centered around what qualifies as a "psychedelic experience," the importance of these classifications becomes less critical in the face of the outcomes delivered. A point worth noting is that from the original definition of a psychedelic experience, this experience is not strictly limited to a class of compounds or dependent upon the ingestion of a specific substance. Many experiences, perhaps life itself, can be classified as psychedelic under these definitions.

Researchers aimed to categorize their psychedelic experience into eleven kinds of phenomena. Participants were given ketamine, LSD, MDMA, and psilocybin in different orders.[45] They discovered that the ratings for LSD, ketamine, and psilocybin were quite similar. There were some differences between the drugs, and ketamine scored the highest on the out-of-body experience. They found MDMA to be more euphoric than profound in a classic sense of psychedelic or mind-enhancing. The rapid antidepressant effects of psilocybin and ketamine are similar.[46]

A recent paper by a well-known ketamine researcher, Dr. Evgeny Krupitsky, reviewed twelve studies in psychedelic administration using psilocybin, ayahuasca, or ketamine and analyzed the association between the mystical experience and symptom reduction in areas as diverse as cancer-related distress, substance use, addiction disorders, and depressive disorders to include treatment-resistant depression.[47] "The association between mystical experience and therapeutic outcome in psychedelic therapy to include ketamine was indicated by most clinical studies in this review. Ketamine is a prescription drug used for general anesthesia, and in sub-anesthetic doses, it induces profound psychedelic experiences and hallucinations."

American soldiers wounded during the Vietnam War were given ketamine anesthesia because of its large margin for safety.[48] In contrast with other anesthetics like opiates, ether, and propofol, ketamine suppresses neither respiration nor heart rate. Most other anesthetics cause profound respiratory depression and require an endotracheal tube in the trachea (windpipe) and a machine to breathe for the patient. Even if one gave a high dose of ketamine, most patients would not stop breathing. Furthermore, ketamine does not depress blood pressure as much as other anesthetics, which is helpful when a wounded soldier loses a lot of blood. Remember that we have only had anesthesia for about 140 years.

The World Health Organization labels ketamine as an essential medication because it requires no supplemental oxygen or medications to support blood pressure and is the most widely utilized anesthetic in the world. Even more, ketamine is safe because it has a high LD50, which stands for "lethal dose in 50 percent of experimental animals tested." This means that you could give a patient very high doses of ketamine, which would not typically result in some physiologic process that kills you. For example, an overdose of fentanyl would kill you by stopping your breathing, or an overdose of Tylenol would poison your liver. All other anesthetics have very low LD50s and will stop you from breathing or suppress your blood pressure to the point of death. Also, there are no withdrawal symptoms after ketamine as with alcohol, benzodiazepines, or opiates. However, excessive doses of ketamine can cause chronic complications. The risk of death after taking ketamine is from intoxication. For example, there have been drownings in bathtubs after ketamine intoxication, similar to alcohol poisoning.

Ketamine has a well-established safety record. This subjective experience, the experiential reality of the ketamine experience, is the strongest argument in favor of classifying ketamine as a psychedelic medicine. Ketamine is and must be considered a psychedelic medicine and included in the clinical repertoire of treating psychiatric illness.

CHAPTER THREE

The Hidden Side of Suicide

"We are always looking for simple answers to complex problems, and they are nearly always wrong."

—H. L. Menken

S uicide is a prominent problem worldwide, and relatively little has been done about it.[1] Staring us in the face is the fact that suicide is not considered a public health crisis; instead, it has been treated as a mental health concern. Even more ominous is that suicide is difficult to study: suicide victims are not available once they have killed themselves. Even if one survives the attempt, they often do not participate in studies, and multiple subjects are needed.

Suicide is one of the leading causes of death globally and has been increasing steadily since the early 2000s in the US; emergency room visits relating to mental-health crises have been rising steadily since 2010 and increased nearly 50 percent during the COVID-19 crisis.[2, 3] In 2018, 10 million people thought about suicide, 3 million planned to commit suicide, 1 million actually attempted suicide, and sadly, close to 800,000 people perished from suicide. Why have so many people contemplated suicide, and why have we seen such an increase? We have no simple answers, but the underpinnings of suicide are invariably multifaceted.

The federal government's commitment to science-based suicide prevention was notably strengthened in 2001 by the National Strategy for Suicide Prevention: Goals and Objectives for Action.[4] Interestingly, suicides have increased despite significant efforts by our governments. Every administration since Nixon has rolled out a suicide prevention program. Perform a search with the name of the US president and "suicide prevention," and you will see nationwide plans for ending suicide. Reagan instituted June as youth suicide prevention month, Bush signed the Garrett Lee Smith Memorial Act, Clinton boosted insurance coverage of mental health services, and Obama signed the Clay Hunt Suicide Prevention Act. Trump signed the law designating 988 as the universal number for the suicide hotline, and Biden expanded the hotline number and awarded millions of dollars to expand mental health services.

Economic downturns almost always bring higher suicide rates compared to prosperous periods.[5, 6] For example, Japan's highest rate of suicide was in 2003, with 34,000 people killing themselves, and that figure fell in 2019 with just over 20,000 suicides. However, in 2020 the number of suicides in Japan is consequential from an industry standpoint; many were young working-class men and women, specifically from the travel industry.[7] Similar trends exist in the US after a crisis.[8, 9]

The 2008 financial crisis resulted in thousands of suicides worldwide. In 2022, according to Daily Wire news, Gustavo Arnal, the fifty-two-year-old chief financial officer of the Bed Bath & Beyond retail chain, jumped to his death from the eighteenth floor of a Manhattan high-rise two days after the struggling company announced plans to slash the jobs of over 6,000 employees and close 150 stores.[10] The stock market, unsurprisingly, experienced historic drops in 2020. We saw millions of jobs lost or furloughed, medical care delayed, and an overwhelming wave of anxiety, fear, and depression. Many Americans fell into poverty for the first time.[11, 12] Over 54 million Americans filed for unemployment, and 60 million European Union jobs were at risk.[13]

Everyone expected a higher suicide rate during and after the first lockdowns because of the mass social trauma.[14] However, the data indicated a short-term decrease in suicides. This is likely due to the "honeymoon period" or the "pulling together phenomenon,"[15, 16] which is defined as a drop in attempted suicide rates initially after a disaster. For example, in the aftermath of the 2011 earthquake and tsunami in Japan, suicide rates in Fukushima, Japan, declined two years following the disaster. Still, the rates increased to pre-disaster levels in the third year.[17] Similar trends existed after the 1918 influenza, SARS, and Ebola epidemics. Several suicidologists believe that the preliminary numbers for suicide deaths may be highly underestimated.[18]

A suicidal person is at war with their brain, and one's situational awareness is flawed. It becomes impossible to discern facts, proof, logic, and concern for yourself. On the battlefield of suicidal ideation, the wounded soldier is in a thick, isolating, never-ending fog. In a very real sense, the person is at war with the mind. When a suicide occurs, the mind wins. The enemy within is trying to ambush the paralyzed mind in the kill zone. The voices telling the mind to take one's own life likely sound rational and even calming. It might even sound like suicide is the best thing for everyone, including yourself. Those voices asking you to drop your defenses. Then, in a moment of intense vulnerability, if a firearm is at hand, just like that, suicide strikes with nearly 99 percent accuracy. Your chances of survival are only slightly improved with other measures. As in a war, the person needs a leader outside one's thinking and limited perception. That leader is intuition. That person may be the one with suicidal ideation, or it might be the parent trying to save their child.

* * * *

Case Study: Dennis Hartman

"This is an incredible story about a man suffering from major refractory depressive disorder his entire life, associated with traumatic stress disorder resulting from childhood abuse. Dennis describes his existence as 'misery' and says, 'Living with my depression feels like pain.' He further explains that it's not something you can show someone, like pointing to an injury or a wound, but it feels like physical pain. Dennis recalls, 'I knew I had a problem by the time I was in seventh grade. I had a very traumatic childhood and spent it in a state of intense fear. By the time I reached adolescence, I had a pretty good idea I couldn't do things as other kids could.' Dennis Hartman spent decades working through a roster of medical treatments for depression. He tried every known depressive therapy (SSRIs, SNRIs, tricyclics, benzodiazepines, etc.); notes Dennis, 'A lot of my energy in life has been spent trying to get relief from this pain. On my worst days, I lost the energy. I didn't have the ability or the strength to inhabit that character anymore . . . I just didn't see any way around it.' In his mid-forties, Hartman decided he would end his life, believing wholeheartedly it was humane and reasonable. He explains, 'There's only so much untreatable suffering that one person can be expected to endure in their lifetime.' He chose a date several months away to get his affairs in order and avoid causing his nephew trauma during school finals. Awaiting his date, he heard of an experimental trial using ketamine to treat depression and PTSD. He applied and was immediately accepted.

'The day I received my infusion, my symptoms were raging; anxiety, anhedonia, and insomnia. They turned on the drip, and I was in a dreamlike state, like a spectator watching my thoughts unfold in front of me. Within fifteen to twenty minutes of the end of the infusion, I knew something was different. They asked me questions to monitor my mood, and I had trouble pinpointing my symptoms.' Dennis knew something was missing within a couple of hours of the infusion. He explains, 'It didn't strike me as a wave of massive relief. It didn't feel like something was added to me, like I had superpowers. I didn't have euphoria. It was a gradual realization over a few hours, something was missing and what was missing was something horrible. If you suffer from lifelong depression, as I have, and it's all you've ever known, it becomes part of your identity. You just feel the world is all about pain, and when I got relief from my first infusion, it was like being emancipated.' Since discovering this treatment, Dennis has become a tireless advocate of ketamine therapy, establishing the Ketamine Advocacy Network to spread awareness of the treatment and connect potential patients with doctors who provide it. As of 2018, over 250 clinics and 1,000 practitioners in the US are now offering ketamine therapy."

Source: Wolfson M.D., Phil. The Ketamine Papers: Science, Therapy, and Transformation *(pp. 293–294). Multidisciplinary Association for Psychedelic Studies.*

* * * *

Intuition is the only thing that can save you from suicide. It is integral to preventing the process leading to the taking of one's own life. Intuition is our most profound intelligence that helps us discern the signs of denial. True intuition is one's inner voice and one's most trusted friend. That gut instinct, which is our intuition, might be what helps you make sense of the paralyzing denial in which your brain is entrenched. The signs of denial are rationalization, justification, minimization, excuse-making, and refusal. It's human nature to use denial to eliminate the discomfort of accepting realities we'd prefer not to acknowledge. This is part of "cognitive dissonance."

We are at the front line of one of the worst mental health crises in history. In science, truth is fundamental. But for many caught up in the throes of suicidal ideation, facts and truth matter not. Intuition is a primary defense; in fact, the root of the word, *intuere,* means to guard and protect.

For many patients, there is no objective proof; the only evidence they have is the seemingly endless depression and isolation. This is not to say that intuition is always correct, but when you or your family are faced with suicide, that inner voice will be your most trusted friend; it's the only thing you may have to overcome an otherwise overwhelming darkness.

Like intuition, denial can feel like a mechanism for survival, but denial actually serves our comfort, our emotional pain, and our emotional calm—and it does so through deceit. Intuition is knowing something without knowing why and without seeing complete evidence, but denial is choosing not to see something when all the evidence is there.

Denial, like intuition, turns out to be a protective mechanism for emotional survival. For example, most parents are in denial their children could be severely depressed or have suicidal ideations. In one study, 75 percent of parents did not realize their adolescent was having recurrent thoughts of death.[19] Another study found that 78 percent of suicidal people denied thoughts of suicide before killing themselves. Denial challenges us to ask ourselves, "What is it I am refusing to see here?"

Suicidal behaviors are complex and hard to detect. Having a psychiatric diagnosis increases the likelihood of suicide. Research shows us that depression is firmly correlated with suicide; an untreated psychiatric illness precedes about 78 percent of suicides.[20] Another critical factor is substance abuse, which is causally related to suicide. Opioid-related deaths from overdoses increased during the COVID-19 crisis. We often don't know if an overdose death was an accident or a suicide; if there is no note, the death is always ruled an overdose.

Suicide is incredibly difficult to study because researchers must try to assemble information about the risk factors via psychological autopsy methods and laboratory tests. Even if the person survives the attempt, they are often unable or unwilling to report the factors leading up to their suicidal behavior. People with mental health problems frequently cannot accurately report the factors influencing their behavior. Many people are unwilling to comment on the factors leading to their behavior. The fear of being institutionalized is one such reason. Also, many believe they do not have a problem or doubt there is anything or anyone who can help them. Many do not want to receive any intervention. Lastly, many in professions such as the military, law enforcement, or medical community members fear disclosing such information for fear of losing their careers. These concerns create real barriers and prevent those at risk from seeking help.

It is essential to distinguish between suicidal ideation, suicidal plans, suicidal attempts, and suicide death. Suicidal ideations are serious thoughts about killing oneself. Suicidal plans are the formulations of an actual plot to kill oneself. Suicidal attempts are self-injurious behavior with the intent to die. Suicide death is the successful result of the final self-injurious action.

Most experience severe depression and suicidal thoughts for the first time in their early twenties, and predicting who will be affected is difficult. Bill Schmitz Jr., former president of the American Association of Suicidology, points out that depression does not have a one-size-fits-all prognosis.[21] "For some, we might prolong life for months, for years. For others, it can be very sudden."

Often, there are no warning signs, and you may wonder what clues you might have missed. Suicide affects men, women, and children, and a multitude of factors drives a person to the decision. Kimberly Van Orden proposed the Interpersonal Theory of Suicide, which purports that the most dangerous form of suicidal desire is caused by the simultaneous presence of thwarted belongingness (I am alone) and perceived burdensomeness (I am a burden).[22] We know that most suicide cases meet the criteria for a psychiatric disorder.[23] When suicidal thoughts occur, the transition to a suicide attempt happens quickly, suggesting the need for rapid intervention. Survivors of suicide attempts often describe the experience as if their brains had been ambushed by their negative internal monologue, which emphasizes the pointlessness of existence.

* * * *

Case Study: Steve

Steve is an aerospace engineer and entrepreneur who loves living life to its fullest. Months prior, he had been involved in a bicycle crash where he sustained a severe traumatic brain injury (TBI) and, as a result, underwent several surgeries. One night, Steve called his physician and asked if he had thirty minutes to talk. He spoke in a concerned and unusual voice, describing the night he attempted suicide. Steve recounted walking furiously through the desert in the middle of the night, and his only mission was to take his own life. He planned to find a place next to a tree and deliberately fall on his knife. Like an engineer, he had envisioned how it would play out for several weeks—where to put the knife in the ground, how to fall on it, and the best time of night he needed to complete his task. He had researched the fastest method of self-exsanguination (bleeding out).

Steve emphasized that he felt he had little control over his suicide attempt. It was as if his brain had hijacked his emotions and began controlling his actions. However, when that final moment in the desert came, he could not bring himself to fall on that knife. In fact, this was Steve's second attempt to take his life, and he nearly succeeded. Steve was experiencing major depression from his TBI. Suicidal behavior is common after major head trauma.

Steve was given ketamine, and his motivation to kill himself subsided. This gave him time to seek help for his depression and traumatic brain injury, and eventually he overcame his condition. Since, he has never had thoughts of suicide.

* * * *

Evolutionary psychiatry teaches us that mother nature cares little if we feel good or bad. At some point in our evolution, we realized that death of the body is the same as the death of the mind, and we became the only animals to desire and choose suicide as mental oblivion.[24] Suicide is a distinctive feature of humankind and to find its reasons, we need to look at how we differ from other species of animals.[25] As twin studies suggest, genetics may play a role in why we commit suicide.[26] Genes are dynamic contributors to our behavioral organization and are sensitive to the feedback systems from our internal and external environments. The selfish gene theory explains that we are inherently programmed to preserve and propagate our existence through our genetic material called DNA.[27] After birth, our behaviors are shaped through the constant interplay between genetic potential and our environment. Emotions, anxiety, and depression all have evolutionary benefits.[28] Today, there is a mismatch between our ancient emotional wiring and how we live in society.

Natural selection shapes our emotions to maximize the survival of the species. We are only about 300 generations removed from our Stone Age ancestors. We can choose to take our own lives, whereas other animals never premeditate the end of their own lives, at least not in the way we think about suicide.

Our human brains enable us to allow or inhibit impulses and emotional reactions, select a choice of behavioral responses, delay gratification, and much more. This prevents us from reacting to impulses from the lower brain, an important human evolutionary advance.

A Brief History of Suicide

The word suicide breaks down into the Latin words *sui* and *caedere*, which together translate to "kill oneself." Suicide and depression have always been omnipresent, and at some stage in evolution, it must have dawned on human beings that the death of the body brings with it the death of the mind.[29] The earliest accounts of suicide and depression appear in Mesopotamia around 2000 BC. Mental illness was viewed as a religious matter, and methods for treating depression included beatings, physical restraints, and starvation to "drive" demons out. The Romans and Greeks had more pragmatic attitudes toward the concept of suicide. In ancient Greece, suicide was considered a disgraceful act. A person thus did not receive the death rites accorded common citizens. Life was a gift, and death was subjected to the will of the gods. In contrast, Christians viewed suicide as a mortal sin, as outlined by St. Thomas Aquinas (c. 1225–1274). "Therefore, killing oneself is contrary to natural inclination and the charity according to which everyone ought to love himself." During a period in early Christianity, if a man committed suicide with a knife, his hand would be cut off and punished separately, and the knife would then be banished and thrown beyond the city walls. The ancient Greeks and Romans introduced the concept that depression and suicide are biologically associated, coining the term "melancholia." Persian physicians wrote about mental illness arising from the brain. They believed melancholy to be caused by an imbalance of body fluids called humors (yellow bile, black bile, phlegm, and blood). Hippocrates believed melancholia was derived from an excess of black bile, and his treatments included bloodletting, baths, exercise, and diet. Along with Hippocrates's treatments, doctors from these times used donkey's milk, leeches, massage, sex, poppy extracts, and meditation.[30]

The medieval mind was caught between the Dark Ages' ignorance and the Renaissance's illumination. Despite advances in medicine, it was still a common belief that demons and the anger of the gods caused depression. During the Middle Ages, Christianity dominated European thinking on mental illness, with people again attributing it to the devil, demons, and witches. During the fifteenth-century Renaissance and into the seventeenth century, public burnings, drownings, and exorcisms were widespread, popularizing the term "lunatic asylums." Many innocent women were burned alive at the stake due to postpartum depression. Ideas about suicide began shifting after the Renaissance period. In the early seventeenth century, Burton, a physician, published *The Anatomy of Melancholy*, outlining the social and psychological causes of depression and suicide, such as fear, loneliness, and poverty.[31] Burton recommended methods to clear toxins from the body through bloodletting, diet, exercise, herbs, music, and travel. Archaic treatments such as water immersion (waterboarding) and centrifugal force (spinning stools) were commonplace.[32]

The period known as "The Enlightenment" promoted changes in medicine and engineering and allowed the first suggestions of psychotherapy. US inventor Benjamin Franklin developed an ancient form of electroshock therapy. By the late 1800s, depression and the act of suicide were thought to be permanent inheritable illnesses rather than moral sins.

Suicide: A Judicial or a Medical Issue?

In many modern societies, suicide and attempted suicide are considered crimes under common law. The successful perpetrator's possessions could be confiscated, and the unsuccessful were imprisoned. The party provoking the suicide, by a love spat, for example, could also face a penalty. In England, attempted suicide was not decriminalized until 1961. In the ten years prior, nearly 6,000 people were prosecuted, of whom 5,400 were found guilty and imprisoned or fined. It was common practice in the 1950s to have a policeman sitting at the bedside of an unconscious person who attempted suicide, waiting to interview them.[33]

In the early 1900s, suicide was illegal and considered a judicial rather than a medical problem, and English law distinguished between suicide and homicide. The following English account of the Ashby case illustrates this point:

On June 25, 1914, in the small coastal town of Lowestoft, England, 59-year-old Louisa Ashby cut her own throat with a razor and lay down on her bed. Her granddaughter discovered her covered in blood and ran to inform her mother that "grandmother had cut her finger." They rushed Louisa to the nearby North Suffolk hospital. The hospital matron requested a police officer stay and take sole charge and responsibility for Ms. Ashby. The matron accused the police of not doing his duty, alleging the woman had committed attempted murder and should be charged. The hospital matron even threatened to take Ashby and put her outside the hospital gates. Louisa Ashby died two days later.

Source: "A history of self-harm in Britain." 2015.[34]

The tragic Ashby case demonstrates how far we have come in recognizing and treating suicide. The idea of "self-harm," as we presently understand it, did not exist in 1914. Terms such as self-cutting, self-mutilation, flesh-picking, and self-biting were not addressed in nineteenth-century writings. In the case of Louisa Ashby, the police were reluctant to charge her with the offense of attempting suicide because that would involve taking responsibility for that person. Suicide and attempted suicide were illegal in England and Wales until 1961, and the 1930 Mental Treatment Act was considered the starting point for integrating general and mental medicine in Britain.[35]

Reasons for Suicide

We can categorize the reasons humans make the choice to die via suicide—mental illness, financial crises, traumatic stress, substance abuse, fear of loss, hopelessness, chronic pain and disease, social isolation, and a "cry for help." Suicidal behavior often presents as hopelessness and worthlessness, not wanting to be a burden to others, or unwillingness to suffer unbearable pain. Many suicidal people speak openly and often about killing themselves.

Mental Illness

The choice to go through with a suicide attempt is often made impulsively, but plotting a suicide attempt involves extensive planning. Nonverbal behavior, isolation, withdrawal, excessive sleeping, substance abuse, increased agitation, and anxiousness are signs that a person may be considering suicide. Unrelenting depression is the most common factor driving a person's decision to prematurely end their life. Depression causes people to feel intense hopelessness, making them unable to see any other way to relieve their emotional pain outside of suicide.

Access to Mental Health Care

Even since the lockdowns ended, we have continued to have inadequate access to mental health care, affecting all ethnicities, men, women, and children. The highest rates of suicide occur in American Indian and Alaskan communities and are due to cultural beliefs and, in part, to a lack of culturally appropriate mental health care.[36] Rural and remote communities have less access to mental health care and experience higher rates of suicide.

Evidence suggests that veteran suicide is partially due to a lack of mental health care providers who can relate to the military and being deployed in the war. The increase in veteran suicides has resulted in many US legislators increasing their funding for "gatekeeper training" programs.[37]

Laypersons could be trained to interact with those at risk for suicide, giving them the means to refer these people to mental health support services. First-aid responders and teachers receive mental-health care training in some states, and gatekeeper training is gaining popularity. For example, Utah has created hotlines that connect callers to licensed mental-health professionals using a smartphone application. Efforts to expand services by federally mandating private insurance to cover mental health have been passed, but the enforcement of these laws is left to the individual states.

Trauma

Adverse childhood trauma and abuse (both physical and sexual) significantly increase the risk of suicide, even years after the actual event.[38] In a survey, nearly one-quarter of those interviewed thought about taking their own life at some point. The diagnosis of PTSD and depression raises suicide risk because depression is common after trauma, and among those with PTSD, feelings of isolation and hopelessness often lead to suicidal behaviors.

Bullying, shaming, and humiliation place children at an increased risk for suicide, especially in LGBTQ adolescent populations. Social media platforms and cyberbullying have compelled many children, adolescents, and adults to take their own lives; when directly or indirectly linked to suicide, this has been referred to as "cyberbullicide."[39, 40]

Substance Abuse, Firearms, and Impulsivity

Half of the United States has experienced an increase in suicides greater than 30 percent, and it is now the second leading cause of death (behind accidents) for those ages 10 to 34.[41] Growing economic disparities, unmet mental health needs, easy access to guns, and the opioid crisis are all partly to blame. Decreasing our inhibitions increases the chance of acting on suicidal ideation. Alcohol and gun sales have significantly increased over the last decade and boomed in 2020, increasing by over 40 and 200 percent respectively.[42] Increasing access to a means of committing suicide will increase the risk of dying in a suicide attempt. Males, especially veterans and police officers, die from suicide more often than women because of firearms.[43]

Hopelessness, Social Isolation, and Fear of Loss

Experiencing prolonged hopelessness and isolation for any reason increases the risk of suicide. Academic failure, lockdowns, loss of social status, financial problems, and the end of a romantic relationship can lead to depression and suicide, as can being arrested or imprisoned. In the book *Talking to Strangers*, Malcolm Gladwell eloquently describes how Sandra Bland, a woman of color, was incarcerated after an escalated altercation with a white police officer during a traffic stop where she failed to use a turn signal. Indications are that she hung herself three days later in her jail cell.[44]

People become socially isolated for many reasons—losing a spouse, partner, or loved one, separation or divorce, physical or mental illness, social anxiety, retirement, or an unfamiliar environment. Those facing social or physical challenges cannot see a path to improve their situation and may resolve to end their life. Many studies cite hopelessness as a common factor contributing to the ultimate decision to commit suicide. When people feel they have lost all hope and cannot change their outlook, this can eclipse the positive aspects of their lives, making suicide seem like an option. Internal factors such as low self-esteem can cause social isolation, leading to loneliness, depression, and suicide. Socially isolated people often use alcohol or drugs to mask their pain, decreasing their inhibitions and increasing their risk of suicide.

Chronic Pain and Disease

People with chronic pain or illness often exhibit suicidal behaviors for many reasons:

Lack of hope or cure;

Loss of autonomy and ability to do enjoyable or meaningful activities;
Disease-related symptoms;
Fear of future suffering;
A lack of reprieve from their suffering.

For many, suicide may seem a viable way to control their suffering and maintain their dignity. Euthanasia, or assisted suicide, is legal in Australia, Belgium, Canada, Columbia, Luxembourg, Netherlands, New Zealand, Spain, and Switzerland. Canada has recently been scrutinized for pushing euthanasia too aggressively. Cancer, neurological disorders, and severe depression commonly account for the majority of assisted suicides. People afflicted with chronic pain and terminal illness often feel they are a burden to family members and friends because they require help with finances, going to the doctor, or household duties. They rationalize that life for those around them would be better if they were gone. This type of internal dialogue is a common warning sign of suicide; it was undoubtedly the rhetoric my grandfather used before killing himself.

Mental illness is a substantial contributor to the global burden of disease. Over 300 million people of all ages suffer from depression worldwide, and the disease is expected to become the leading cause of disability by 2030.

A Cry for Help

People sometimes want to show the world and those around them how much they are suffering. These are not suicide attempts per se but are a cry for help. Some engage in these acts not because they wish to die, but because they don't have a discernible path to help. Unfortunately, these cries for help can end fatally if the person misjudges the lethality of the chosen method, as often happens with medications. One example is Brandi Bielicki's story about her ten-year-old daughter's suicide (see the chapter on adolescent suicide).

Psychology Theories of Suicide

The theories around the psychology of suicide are essential to understand as they give a glimpse into the subtle signs of a person who is suicidal. There are two general types of psychological factors that convey vulnerability to suicide risk. First, subjectively reported psychological and temperamental factors such as depressive personality traits, impulsiveness, aggressiveness, or hopelessness about the future predict vulnerability to suicide risk. Second, neurocognitive factors such as difficulty with decision-making, problem-solving, cognitive control, and verbal fluency also convey suicide risk.

Cognitive theories of suicidal behaviors are based on well-validated peer-reviewed research. The interpersonal-psychological theory of suicidal behavior suggests that completed suicides require three specific characteristics:

1. A sense of thwarted belongingness
2. A sense of burdensomeness
3. A gained capability for suicide

Suicide is not simply a bout of severe depression. Instead, it is a severe depression in people with a particular moment of extreme vulnerability combined with a readily available means to end their lives.

Suicidal patients pay close attention to environmental cues that are specifically related to their suffering, particularly the sense of hopelessness, burdensomeness, and loneliness, causing extreme difficulty in finding solutions to their problems.

Fear of death has a protective effect in preventing suicide. According to suicide expert Dr. John Mann, even in extreme cases, fear of death stops most suicides. The role of the amygdala, an almond-shaped structure in the brain, is crucial in suicide because it controls impulsivity, fear, suicidal thoughts, anxiety, and depression.[45] It is also the same part of the brain affected by attention deficit disorder. The amygdala's function is to process emotions and make decisions, the two keystones of suicide. When this fear inhibition is removed, and the person is no longer indecisive, suicide may occur, and this is exactly what happens when a person jumps from the Golden Gate Bridge. The four-second fall ends with the victim hitting the waters of the San Francisco Bay at seventy-five miles per hour. Many die instantly from internal injuries, while others drown or die from hypothermia. Since the Golden Gate Bridge opened in 1937, there have been over 1,700 suicides.[46, 47]

The amygdala processes fear and threatening stimuli and thus plays a prominent role in someone contemplating suicide. Early studies in the 1960s on the amygdalae of wild monkeys are fascinating (and grim) and clearly demonstrate what happens when the amygdala is altered. Traveling to an uninhabited island near Puerto Rico, Dr. Arthur Kling captured a group of wild monkeys and then took the animals back to the lab.[48] Dr. Kling performed brain surgery on the monkeys, making cuts into the amygdalae. When he released them back into the jungle, what he described was horrific but genuinely extraordinary. The monkeys had trouble navigating their surroundings, and some starved to death. Many could not recognize which animals were prey and which were predators and were devoured. In the river, others could no longer sense the danger of rapids and were taken away and drowned. Many displayed no fear of an approaching troop and were subsequently killed and dismembered. Dr. Kling also kept some of the animals in the lab. The amygdala lesioned females mishandled, bit, and killed their newborn babies shortly after birth. The mother behaved like the infant was a strange object to be mouthed, bitten, and tossed around.

In the words of Lord Byron, indeed, sometimes fact is stranger than fiction. Humans are sometimes born with a destroyed amygdala. One such famous case is that of S.M., also sometimes referred to as SM-046. She was born with Urbach-Wiethe disease, a genetically inherited disorder that results in complete amygdalae destruction. The media dubbed her as the "woman with no fear." Experiments with S.M. revealed no fear in response to snakes, spiders, and a haunted hospital called the Waverly Hills, which is popularized as one of the "scariest places on earth." However, one experience elicited fear in S.M. as outlined in the book *Breathe* by James Nestor. She was administered breaths of 35 percent carbon dioxide in a medical experiment and experienced a full-fledged panic attack, fearful of being drowned.[49] Science is often more complex than we comprehend.

Sometimes the reasons a person kills themself are only revealed after their death. Autopsies on suicide victims reveal that over 90 percent have a diagnosable mental disorder at the time of death, though some have debated this.[50] The presence of mental illness is among the most consistently reported risk factors for suicidal behavior. For example, a history of major depression is one of the strongest predictors of suicidal ideation, but it does not predict actual suicide attempts. Therefore, it's important to distinguish between suicidal ideation and suicide attempts. Even more perplexing is the evidence that most people with mental health disorders never attempt suicide.

People with a family history of mental disorders and suicidal behavior may have an increased risk for suicidal behavior. A family history of panic disorder, antisocial personality disorder, and suicidal behavior may predict suicidal behavior among offspring.[51] Indeed, having a first-degree relative who committed suicide predicts more than twice the probability of the offspring killing themselves.[52] Relating genetic factors to suicidal behaviors is promising, but it is difficult to reproduce these initial findings.

Many scientists highlight that the environment plays more of a role than genetics. Current research shows a strong association with the environmental regulation of genes that play a role in the human stress response system.[53] Since you cannot choose your parents, knowing that a person with a family history of mental disorders can overcome these difficulties through positive environmental factors and close, productive relationships is essential.

Childhood trauma, such as sexual and physical abuse, often leads to suicidal behavior. Shared genetic and neuro-biological characteristics may explain the parent and offspring link.[54] Especially when combined with a history of childhood abuse, parents who are impulsive and aggressive are more likely to have children who are impulsive and aggressive. Both familial transmissions of sexual abuse and impulsive aggression are potential mediators in the genetic transmission of suicidal behavior. Even studies of nonhuman primates reveal that early infant experiences such as maternal deprivation contribute independently to developing impulsive, aggressive, and self-injurious behavior.

A history of suicidal behavior is the strongest predictor of future suicide attempts and suicide death. People who have previous suicide attempts are nearly 40 times more likely to die by suicide than those without such a history. Multiple suicide attempts are associated with an increased risk of subsequent suicidal behavior and often do so with increasing severity. So, if you have ever wondered why a nurse or a doctor routinely asks you if you are suicidal or have ever attempted suicide, this is why.

Using New Technology to Detect Suicidality

For over a century, psychiatrists have evaluated patients by asking them about their lives, and while they are talking, the doctor will carefully observe their speech and behavior. However, people with suicidal ideation often consciously or unconsciously hide their emotions. Tools are being produced that may change this model. Social media has built an entire industry predicting a person's behavior based on smartphone use and online activity. Our Internet searches and social media history are time-stamped and digitized, effectively leaving a breadcrumb trail of our thoughts and emotions. Psychiatrists are using this data to measure and evaluate our mental states as it may have extraordinary potential for psychiatric diagnosis and treatment of mental disorders.

Rosemary Sedgewick wrote a piece in *Current Opinions in Psychiatry* titled "Social media, internet use and suicide attempts in adolescents." Studies have shown that the words we use to express ourselves on social media can predict psychosis.[55] Speech and facial recognition technologies can be used by a psychiatrist during a session to precisely measure a patient's expression, the words they use, and the intonation of their voice. Such tools can recognize the subtle changes that occur when a patient becomes psychotic. For example, the frequency of possessive pronouns can predict with an accuracy of 83 percent whether someone is at risk for psychosis, and decreased facial expressivity may predict suicide. App-based therapies allow doctors to better connect with patients.[56] Using artificial intelligence to quantify large amounts of data will help psychiatrists discover insights that are not necessarily intuitive.[57]

Matthew Nock, a Harvard psychologist and a MacArthur Genius Award winner has made advances in detecting suicide risk. He uses tools that examine unconscious bias, known in research as implicit association tests (IAT). An IAT test may show a series of pictures or words associated with death (suicide, gunshot, hanging, die, deceased, death) or life (alive, thrive, breathing, living) paired with pronouns or words related to self or other (I, myself, mine, they, themselves, their). A computer gives the test and asks subjects to sort the word pairs into categories associated with life or death. Many studies have shown that suicidal patients, even those who deny intent, have faster reaction times for pairs linking self-injury or death and self. The effect is so robust that Nock and his team have developed a computer game to train patients to dissociate the connection between self-injury or death and self.

Malcolm Gladwell eloquently illustrates suicidality in his book, *Talking to Strangers*.[58] He points out that suicide is closely tied to the physical environment: when we look at a person apart from their circumstances, we cannot see their whole story. Instead, we need to be looking at the entire picture, in a broader cultural and environmental context. Suicide is multifaceted, and people get to that endpoint in many ways. Suicide might seem like a real solution to an immediate problem. They view their situation as a mechanical or engineering problem and see specific methods of how to ultimately fix it.

Gladwell highlights the example of suicide rates in 1960s Britain coupled with the availability of the commonly used "town gas." After the Second World War, many British homes were heated using "town gas," a deadly mixture of hydrogen, methane, carbon dioxide, and carbon monoxide.[59] During this time, "town gas" suicide victims were frequently found with their heads wrapped in a blanket or a coat and a tube underneath pumping out the gas. Nearly 6,000 people committed suicide in Britain in 1962, with 2,500 using the town gas method. Pulitzer Prize-winning poet Sylvia Plath was perhaps the most well-known case of this type of suicide.

Plath struggled with depression her entire life. The night of her suicide, she left some food and water in her children's room, opened their bedroom window, then affixed a paper containing only four words, "Please call Dr. Horder," on the baby carriage, and concealed the gap around the kitchen door with towels. Turning on the gas of her kitchen stove, she placed her head inside the oven as far as possible, fell asleep from the carbon monoxide, and so took her own life.

The Sylvia Plath example shows the phenomenon of coupling as it relates to suicide. Plath constantly wrote about suicide and attempted it many times. People are not actively looking to kill themselves. Rather, they have a reason to believe that by killing themselves they can escape from pain. When people are looking for a way to kill themselves, not just any method will do. Plath had all her conditions met at a vulnerable moment, and she died the way she wrote about it in her poems. In the example of Sylvia Plath, the method of using "town gas" was right there in front of her and fit all her requirements: with the ultimate result being death, it was clean with no grotesque mess, and she could lie in an unchanged state. It was said Plath went out "in a woman's way."

CHAPTER FOUR

Suicide and Depression in Children and Adolescents

"The pandemic may have been a perfect storm, but we've all been in very different boats."
—Paul Nestadt MD, *Johns Hopkins University Psychiatrist*

"I want to kill myself," announced the Jefferson Elementary School students to their counselor, Olivia Carter: some as young as eight years old, in Cape Girardeau, Missouri. Carter started working there in 2016 and seldom remembers using the school suicide protocol. Nowadays, it's one a month. She often answers questions like, "What happens when you die?" She feels a good number of the kids understand what it means to end their life by suicide.[1]

An unimaginable array of factors must come together, precipitating a child to reach a point of desperation and arrive at the conclusion that taking their own life is the best option. It's uncomfortable to think our youth are thinking about death, dying, and even contemplating suicide, but it's happening. One thing is clear: if suicide is successful, opportunities for treatment, relief, and hope are no longer possible.

Most parents are astounded to learn their child is contemplating suicide or self-harm.[2] One study found that parents and caregivers were unaware their children had tried to kill themselves in 88 percent of cases. The signs of suicide in adolescents are subtle and much different than in adults.

Suicide and Depression in Children and Adolescents

Young people are hurting. Today, youths with no prior history of mental health disorders are unexpectedly contemplating suicide. The National Alliance on Mental Illness reports that nearly 20 percent of high school students say they've had serious thoughts of suicide, and 9 percent have attempted to take their lives. In this century, suicide is the second leading cause of death between the ages of 10 to 14 and the third leading cause between the ages of 15 to 24. In 1983, suicide ranked as the eighth leading cause of death for persons 15 to 24 years old.[3]

From 1900 to the 1950s, the youth suicide rate was flat, then beginning in 1955, the rate began to climb.[4] Then the youth suicide rate remained stable between 1950 to 1980. Then from the 1980s to now, something changed and rates increased dramatically. Undoubtedly, these rates have varied with the means of suicide available, pandemics, wars, and financial crises.[5] The old saying "trust your gut" refers to trusting these feelings of intuition. Right now, those uncomfortable feelings of your gut sinking beg the question we should all be asking ourselves: what are kids fearing today that they did not fear twenty years ago?

According to the MNIH, 4 million adolescents aged 12 to 17 experienced major depression in 2020.[6] The CDC tracks emergency room visits for self-harm, making it an objectively measured behavior and, therefore, not subject to self-reported bias. Among girls aged 10 to 14, self-harm has quadrupled in the last twelve years. Depression, suicidal thoughts, and self-harm are well documented in teenagers, but less attention has been paid to young children.[7, 8]

Things are not getting better for our children despite massive efforts by our governments. In the US, depression and mood disorders are rampant, and we have become quite comfortable, even satisfied, putting our children on psychotropic medications. Over 25 percent of children are on mental health medications.[9, 10] Attention deficit hyperactivity disorder or ADHD has significantly increased in the last fifteen years, seemingly more in the US than in Europe and mainly in children.[11] Correspondingly, the number of prescriptions written for ADHD medications also increased. The annual number of antidepressants prescribed has tripled over the past two decades, and the pandemic undoubtedly pushed this number upwards.

The impact of lockdowns on children, with and without mental illness, reaches beyond imagination. A survey by Young Minds revealed that 80 percent of young people with mental illness reported worsening their condition because of lockdown measures.[12] Lockdowns aggravate underlying problems, such as parental pressure, parental scolding, household discord, domestic violence, substance abuse, access to firearms, and the inability to escape abusive environments.[13] The president of the American Association of Suicidology, Jonathan Singer, says, "It's probably going to be worse for those who were already struggling or disadvantaged by society. Little kids essentially lost a year of socialization." Perhaps we should take a step back and consider the reasons why an association of suicidology is needed.[14, 15]

Former CDC director Dr. Robert Redfield highlighted that over 7 million kids in the US get mental health services at schools. The curtailing of in-person counseling has negatively affected our youth with mental health disorders as we watch drug use and suicide increase in adolescent individuals.[16] Even more troublesome, UNICEF warned that 1.2 million children could die from malaria, pneumonia, and diarrhea because of the economic impact of lockdowns in developing countries.[17] It's important to mention the following:[18]

- The increase in human trafficking for sexual exploitation
- A surge in child labor and forced marriage
- An increase in school dropouts
- A reduction in household income and savings
- Food and ration shortages, all during the lockdowns
- Increased mental health problems such as trauma, anxiety, depression, and despair
- An increase in child suicide, especially in poor communities

The mental health crisis has perhaps taken a heavier emotional and psychological toll on young people than on adults with acute mental-health emergencies, and youth suicide rates are increasing to alarming levels. Youth suicides pre- and post-pandemic were counted in fourteen US states. The finding confirmed what many had been predicting all along—that the mental health crisis would be worse for children and adolescents than adults. Georgia, Indiana, New Jersey, Oklahoma, Virginia, and California had an increase in children killing themselves; Nevada also had a similar increase.[19]

If you need more convincing that we have a youth mental illness crisis, read about the increase in emergency department and hospital admissions in 2020. One spokesperson for the Muir Medical Center in Walnut Creek, California, reported that they've seen "a year's worth of youth suicide attempts in just four weeks." This data reflects the highest proportion of suicidal adolescents ever recorded.[20] *The Journal of Pediatrics* cited a concerning increase in hospital admissions for children with suicidal ideation, which increased by 57 percent between pre-pandemic 2019 and 2020.[21] The Children's Hospital Association reported the number of children ages 6 to 12 who visited children's hospitals for suicidal thoughts or self-harm had more than doubled between 2016 (2,555) and 2021 (5,485).[22]

Rates of youth suicidal ideation have drastically increased in pediatric emergency departments. A recent *Lancet Psychiatry* study highlighted that 8 percent of children ages 9 to 10 reported suicidal thoughts, and 2 percent initiated an actual suicide attempt.[23] A CDC study showed that emergency departments are treating more and more children per day for mental health conditions. At the Riley Hospital for Children in Indianapolis, the number of children and teens hospitalized after suicide attempts went up from 67 in 2019 to 108 in 2020. Children's Hospital of Oakland reported a 66 percent increase in 10- to 17-year-olds screening positive for suicidal ideation in the emergency department. Intermountain Mental Health Services have reported a 25 percent increase in mental-health referrals.

Socioeconomic factors may heavily contribute to suicide, especially among minority ethnic groups. A 2016 study found that children aged 5 to 11 who died by suicide were more likely to be African Americans and males.[24, 25] Similar data exists for other minority groups.

The mental health crisis may be to blame for the increase in youth suicide, but the crisis has been going on for a long time. The pandemic has exposed the longstanding shortcomings of the mental health system. Even before 2020, encounters of suicidal ideation and attempts in US children and adolescents more than doubled between 2008 and 2015, and half of these resulted in hospitalization. The observed increases matched the increasing prevalence of depression and mood disorders in the US.[26]

Nurse and single mom Brandi Bielicki experienced how deadly a mental-health crisis can be for a child.[27] Ms. Bielicki saw no signs her daughter, Kodie, felt suicidal. Kodie was an easygoing child and very close to her mom. She left no clues in her diary or text messages at school or home. Bielicki recalls, "One day, Kodie called me to say that she lost a tooth." When Brandi returned home, her daughter's door was open, and the authorities later found her body in a nearby field with a short note. Kodie had taken a lethal amount of medication.[28] Brandi believes her daughter did something "super-impulsive"; a ten-year-old does not understand the permanence of their actions, nor do they even know help is available. Utah passed a law this year requiring that elementary schools begin offering suicide-prevention programs. We urgently need programs like this because many schools only have one counselor for roughly every 250 students.

Rodney Moore Sr. of Anaheim, California, lost his fourteen-year-old son, Rodney Jr., to suicide in January 2021.[29] Mr. Moore believes his son despaired when his school did not reopen. He explains, "Rodney Jr.'s grades started dropping with distance learning. His world changed." Rodney Jr. was an active teenager who adored animals and playing his saxophone. Adriana Moore, Rodney's mother, noted that he kept on saying, "I don't see the point. Nothing's going to get better." Rodney's parents felt their son was deeply affected and depressed, but they never suspected that it was to such a degree he would take his own life. Mrs. Moore exclaims, "You should never have to say goodbye to your kids. Every time we close our eyes, we see how we found him." Rodney Sr. adds, "Although the coronavirus didn't take my son's life directly, it took it indirectly."

Despite parents' protests, most school districts decided not to reopen in 2020. A Baltimore family said the school shutdowns were devastatingly impacting children. After their fourteen-year-old son, Michael Myronyuk, took his own life, they blamed the isolation and depression secondary to the effects of the lockdowns.[30] In December 2020, an eleven-year-old boy in Woodbridge, California, killed himself with a firearm during a Zoom class. In Arizona, the Pima school district in Tucson reported two student suicides in 2020, while the Vail district reported three.[31] A Maine teenager took his life in December 2020, his father attributing his son's suicide to the isolation of the lockdowns.

On April 17, 2020, twelve-year-old Hayden Hunstable took his own life just four days before his thirteenth birthday. His father, Brad Hunstable, made a video two days after he buried his son in their hometown of Aledo, Texas. With hundreds of millions of views, the video garnered considerable attention and exposed the adolescent suicide crisis during the lockdowns. Hayden enjoyed playing football and hanging out with his friends. Before his death, he became consumed by the video game Fortnite. The Hunstables created a foundation in their son's name as a public-service-announcement campaign aimed at educating kids and parents on responsible gaming and parental oversight. The foundation's goal is to pass legislation federally mandating resilience classes as core curriculum for K–12 schools (www.haydenscorner.org).[32]

The Las Vegas Youth Suicide Crisis

Former CDC director Dr. Robert Redfield warned that a rise in adolescent suicides would be one of the most substantial public-health consequences of school closings.[33, 34] On November 11, 2020, then Nevada governor Steve Sisolak opened his virtual town hall meeting with the announcement that another Clark County School District (CCSD) child, this one nine years old, had committed suicide the prior evening. The cause of death was likely asphyxiation. This was the fourth child suicide in a six-week period.[35] The CCSD experienced a cluster of eighteen student suicides between March 16 and December 31, 2020. There was only one student suicide in the CCSD in 2019.

The *New York Times* interviewed CCSD superintendent Jesus Jara who argued for reopening schools, claiming isolation during the lockdowns was to blame for the student suicides.[36] Clark County, Nevada, has one of the highest youth suicide rates in the nation. An online early warning system called GoGuardian, which monitors student's mental-health episodes, sent over 3,000 alerts in 2020 to CCSD officials, raising alarms about suicidal thoughts and self-harm.

A Las Vegas counselor at Shadow Ridge High School told the story of one of her longtime students. This student had overcome much during the 2019–2020 school year, being homeless, living in parks, and working at McDonald's around his school schedule. Two weeks before graduation, the counselor emailed him to say how proud she was of his accomplishments, only to learn that he had recently killed himself with a firearm.

On November 9, 2020, the grandfather of a twelve-year-old boy with no history of mental problems received a call from the CCSD alerting him that the boy was possibly going to commit suicide. At 10:00 p.m., his father discovered him in his room with a noose around his neck constructed from multiple shoestrings and aborted the suicide attempt. The boy searched the internet on "how to make a noose" using his school-issued iPad. The CCSD monitoring program, GoGuardian, detected the boy's search activity and alerted the school, who called the boy's grandfather. His parents asked, "Why?" The boy's only response was "I miss my friends" and "I don't have friends." The boy's dog died during the pandemic, but he was otherwise doing well in virtual school. The grandfather said that his grandson was "Zoomed out" and believes the lockdowns caused the suicide attempt and that being in the classroom even a few days a week might have helped him. He says his grandson has a hard time functioning in isolation.[37]

Las Vegas family therapist, Dr. Sheldon Jacobs, author of the book *48: An Experimental Memoir on Homelessness*, works with CCSD students and parents in the community. He believes the pandemic exacerbated the mental health crisis leading to increases in isolation, anxiety, depression, suicide, and PTSD. The kids he works with are struggling from a lack of social interaction with peers. With many athletic facilities closed during the lockdowns, outlets such as sports were no longer available, and the kids found themselves at home eating more and gaining weight as well as straining their relationships with parents and siblings. He also mentions it's clear the suicide crisis has hit African Americans a lot harder than others in many states. He quotes a study published in *JAMA Psychiatry* that analyzed the records from 1,079 Maryland residents who died from suicide during the peak of the lockdowns and found African American suicides doubled compared to previous years.[38, 39] Most of the suicides have been minorities of lower socioeconomic status, which he says is following the national trend; minority groups face unique economic challenges and losing a job or a loved one might be felt even more intensely by these communities.

Veteran Las Vegas school teacher Louie Amelburu has taught health education and suicide prevention for over thirty years in a high-risk middle school. He says, "Youth suicide has always been a problem in Las Vegas, ever since I can remember, and it's like the same thing happens every year, and it never changes." He agrees the lockdowns are fueling the isolation and depression of kids, but he points out that kids are constantly on their phones, looking for recognition and attention. He says that when kids do not get the love and attention they need at home, they will find it elsewhere. Enter social media. Amelburu highlights that the internet has provided a way for kids to get how-to descriptions for suicide and lethal means to kill themselves and sometimes others. "What the social media world has done to teenage girls is damn near unbearable," Amelburu says. It has spearheaded the narcissistic, self-aggrandizing element of a social media presence.

Mr. Amelburu describes the rhetoric on social media such as Twitter and Facebook as "processed words." Just like "processed food" is bad for us, he believes that "processed words" are equally bad and contribute to stress, especially during lockdowns. Finally, Mr. Amelburu sees many kids who have decreased daily physical activity and substantial weight gain. His observations are valid. In the 1960s, less than 5 percent of kids were obese and today, nearly 50 percent of kids entering high school are overweight.[40] We all know a physically active lifestyle benefits mental health. At the end of our interview, we agreed that suicide is preventable. Teachers, parents, and school counselors must stand ready to screen for student suicide risk and be willing to provide immediate support.

Amelburu explains that kids are very impulsive, and many have attention problems; chronic insomnia and stress lead to impulsivity and fear. He teaches adherence to structure because that provides comfort for his students. The part of the brain responsible for impulse control is the tiny pecan-shaped amygdala (discussed in chapter 3); it also serves as the central processor for fear and stores short-term information. In fact, many medications designed to treat attention deficit disorder (ADD) stimulate the amygdala. Sleep deprivation, even for short periods, disrupts transmission of messages to and from the amygdala, leading to impulsivity and learning difficulties. We store fear learning and fear memories in the prefrontal cortex, which communicates directly with the amygdala.

Researchers debate the pros and cons of the effects of social media on psychological well-being.[41, 42] Psychologists Jonathan Haidt and Jean Twenge have been tracking the attitudes and behaviors of teens for years.[43, 44] They observed a sudden uptick in teens and young adults expressing depression, hopelessness, self-harm, and suicide in 2012. Before the pandemic, they wrote that the rates of depression among adolescents had nearly doubled. Their research has shown that teens have given up most of their social lives to their phones, spending less time with their friends in person, communicating more electronically, and using social media. Teens were becoming unhappy and depressed at precisely the time that smartphones were becoming ubiquitous. By 2020, Haidt wrote that more than 25 percent of female teenagers had major depression, whereas the comparable number is 9 percent for boys.

A recent study highlighted that when adults gave up Facebook for just four weeks, subjective well-being and happiness increased, and they were less lonely and depressed.[45] Instagram's popularity strongly affected girls and young women, with many posts re-edited until they were closer to "perfection" than reality. Many counselors and teachers point to children being engulfed in cell phones and social media. Many elementary school children already have cell phones and stay up late checking their phones and social media, resulting in poor sleep.[46, 47] Dr. Twenge asserts that even if the phones are turned off in the room, a child unconsciously knows it's there and its presence can disrupt sleep.[48, 49]

The consequences of social media have been severe, with teen depression doubling since around 2010. When social media became ubiquitous, loneliness and anxiety increased. In the age of social media and intense comparison, students are obsessing about keeping up or achieving unrealistic goals of perfection. This is especially evident among young adolescent girls.

Many of these concerns have been addressed in Jonathan Haidt's book, *The Coddling of the American Mind.*

Dana Gentry, a Las Vegas native who writes for the *Nevada Current*, published an article about the youth suicide crisis in Las Vegas. She wrote that the youth suicides were not because of the pandemic but that it was a normal year for youth suicides and highlighted that Nevada's children were killing themselves at a rate higher than youth in any other state in the nation. She discussed her viewpoints in an interview with me. Gentry says, "It's true that before COVID-19, suicide took the lives of more 12- to 19-year-olds in Nevada than any other cause of death." In 2019, 41 youths in Nevada died by suicide compared to 43 in 2020. But, unlike in 2019, most of the children who committed suicide in 2020 did not have a long-standing history of mental problems; they were regular students. When Ms. Gentry was questioned about the cluster of recent student suicides in the CCSD, she said she had no explanation, but felt it was not because of the pandemic, but rather the mental-health care system, labor market, and justice system exposed by the stress of the pandemic. Suicide is complex, involving layers of risk factors.

Kerala, a small city in India, initially won worldwide praise for its handling of the COVID-19 situation.[50] However, Kerala's success with the pandemic was short-lived because what resulted was horrific: 173 children ages 10 to 18 died by suicide during the lockdowns. The reasons for the suicides seemed minor: routine disciplining by parents for skipping online classes or playing games on smartphones. The isolation caused by the lockdowns also made children overly sensitive to minor domestic issues. In many cases, children spent the time outside of online classes in front of the TV and the internet, leading to psychosocial problems like addiction, lower self-esteem, and decreased interest in physical activities.

A more recent example is the CDC's 2021 report that adolescent hospitalizations were increasing during COVID-19.[51, 52] Again, the media highlighted the dangers of COVID-19 infections and adolescents, which had been very low since the start of the crisis.[53] In this instance, the media failed to report that over 20 percent of those hospitalizations were for psychiatric emergencies, not COVID-19 infections. News reporting agencies have followed a potentially dangerous narrative, especially in people with mental health conditions.

Addressing Suicide with Children and Adolescents

Addressing children's psychological needs is complex, and they need professional help to avert disastrous consequences, such as depression or suicide. Even for adults, suicides are impulsive and unpredictable, and finding a specific cause is challenging. This begs the question, what are the telltale signs for these troubled youth? Depression and self-harm do not appear the same in young children as in teens and adults. Children are more likely to draw pictures or tell a friend about suicidal thoughts, and they may also appear less interested in playing outside or with others. Children who are emotionally withdrawn or depressed should immediately receive psychiatric help. Prominent warning signs for parents that a child may be considering or thinking about suicide are:

- An increase in irritability
- Withdrawal from activities
- A lack of engagement in activities, especially with friends
- Problems with concentration
- Changes in eating and sleeping patterns
- Addiction to video games or any substances
- Gives away possessions
- Makes out a will
- Jokes about committing suicide
- Sends despairing texts or posts online about suicide
- Shows signs of major depression
- Engages in risky behaviors

Veteran suicide prevention specialist and psychiatrist Marc Goulston explains that a suicidal adolescent sees the world as black and white, cold, and deprived. This is meaningful because the adolescent must have a level of trust that they can be heard. If you are a parent worried about your teen having depression or possibly suicidal thoughts, he advises against a heart-to-heart talk unless they initiate it. For many teens, it is like nails on a chalkboard, and they do not respond well. Alternatively, Dr. Goulston suggests bringing up the subject during an activity together.

How Children Experience Suicide

Experiencing the death of a loved one, especially a parent, is the most disruptive and stressful event a child can experience. Approximately 1 in 20 adolescents loses someone to suicide annually, and roughly 1 in 5 does so before reaching adulthood. Common grief reactions include crying, sadness, guilt, and longing. Although the grief following any death may be similar, some features may be more pronounced after a suicide. Crying is usually a good thing; it means they find relief, the hormone oxytocin is surging, and they are not feeling alone.

Parental suicide during adolescence sometimes results in anxiety, depression, and substance abuse; long-term developmental competencies, such as educational and work aspirations, are often diminished in the aftermath. Death differentiates children from their peers. Characteristic reactions in adolescents grieving a loved one lost to suicide include feelings of shock, sadness, guilt, injustice, anger, betrayal, questions of "why," and worrying over the impact of the death on others. For most, the death seems incomprehensible, and it changes the family equilibrium and the ability to support each other.

For a child, death by suicide is the most confusing way to lose someone. The grief following a suicide is experienced more like a death of a traumatic or homicidal nature by adolescents and adults alike. Subtle triggers unrelated to the death or the deceased person (e.g., a song on the radio) can ambush the bereaved adolescent. One child remarked, "when you lose someone through suicide and when you're a kid, you don't really know what's going on. You are so confused because you're just left with so many questions, 'Why,' 'What if,' and 'How?'" For most young people, the bereavement of a suicide or other traumatic death is a new and radical experience for which they have not yet developed a language. One mom said, "My daughter couldn't say how she was feeling, and all she could say was, 'I have feelings.'" They look, sound, and seem to be the same person they were before, but they're not, because while they've experienced the same loss as you, they've experienced it differently.

Treatment of Children and Adolescents for Suicidal Ideation

Suicide is a leading killer of our children in the US, and depression is often resistant to current medical models. Children and adolescents hospitalized for suicidal attempts usually receive psychotherapy, sedating medications, and are often put in restraints. Suicidal adolescents have no choice but to live in hospital psychiatric wards while being treated. When they present to the ED with suicidal ideations, the child is assessed and given a referral for outpatient treatment.

Novel treatments for adolescent suicidality are desperately needed. Despite the number of children receiving mental health treatment, as we've seen, the rates of suicidal ideation are rising. US Surgeon General, Vivek Murthy MD, stated in December 2021 that "One in three high school students reported persistent feelings of sadness or hopelessness, while suicide rates for young people rose 57% in a decade." Major efforts have been dedicated to treating suicidal ideation and self-injurious behavior, but these have only had a small impact. When a child commits suicide, the signs are subtle, the action is impulsive, and it often happens without warning. Most children with suicidal ideation are hospitalized and sedated with medications. Apart from psychiatric care, there is not much out there for treating these desperate children apart from institutionalizing them for their protection. Admitting children to the hospital or a psychiatric facility is problematic because of the anxiety of being away from their parents or other loved ones. And even in the best institutions, the environment is often very stressful. Furthermore, there is often limited availability in mental health facilities, so a patient may have to stay for weeks in a hospital or not be institutionalized at all.

Gavin de Becker's book *The Gift of Fear* perfectly illustrates intuition's true meaning and value.[54] Intuition will save you and your loved ones from the wretchedness of depression and suicide. Western society favors logical, grounded, explainable thought processes that end in supportable explanations, whereas intuition may save your child's or your own life. Trust your intuition when you observe the subtle signs of mental illness or realize that a child could take his or her own life. Some prefer to remain in the comfortable illusion that adolescent suicide is rare, but if you know better, you may be able to save a life.

Treating kids for suicidal ideation comes with limited options, and parents would do anything possible to stop their kids from committing suicide. Naturally, first-line treatment should be any intervention that prevents the child from taking their life. But since ketamine works in adults to stop suicidal ideation, why wouldn't it work for children and adolescents? Several studies on treating children and adolescents with ketamine exist, but we need more in order for it to become a mainstream practice.

Treating children with ketamine for suicidal ideation is a logical choice if it provides time for the parents to get help.[55] Again, the cries to wait for the research will be loud, especially when children are concerned. However, performing research on suicidal adolescents is complex. The studies out there today clearly demonstrate the potential role of ketamine in treating children and adolescents with treatment resistant depression.[56] A case report in 2018 described the successful use of a ketamine infusion in a fourteen-year-old for depression and neuropathic pain.[57] A review of the available studies on the use of ketamine in children and adolescents with psychiatric disorders showed an overall benefit.[58] Lori Calabrese successfully treated suicidal adolescents as young as fourteen in her study. Ongoing studies have found ketamine can lower symptoms in severely depressed teenagers. Ketamine has been safely used for over fifty years in children for anesthesia and sedation. Hopefully, ongoing studies will show that psychedelics like ketamine can help children in severe mental distress, giving society a clearer path to quashing the mental health crisis and these senseless acts of child suicide.[59]

Children learn by example. They can see the hardships and economic effects on the family. When they see their parents stressed out, they are likely to follow. Parents need to play a more proactive role in their children's well-being. Adults are better prepared to deal with stress, whereas children are more likely to break down under pressure, especially during a crisis. Children will be more secure when they observe their parents handling a situation maturely and in a positive frame of mind. We have become a frighteningly lonely society and have taught our children that discomfort is a bad thing and should be avoided at all costs. Children who face difficulties become more resilient. Keeping children away from reality will not shelter them from danger; instead, they should learn by taking the bull by the horns with adult guidance. Parents and guardians should provide an environment of trust, encouraging them to share their fears and insecurities.

Honesty, thinking, and speech are complex processes; thought is the internal dialogue between you and your inner self. This highlights the importance of parents, friends, and family; you can count on them and receive an honest answer that helps you rectify the internal dialogue. One reason criminals in prison rarely get better and instead revert to crime is that they have no choice but to fall on the corrupted dialogue they have cemented into their minds due to a lack of friends and family.

A happy childhood lays the foundation for a bright and secure future. A loving, positive relationship is most important, and the scars left by the pandemic, too, shall pass. However, it is vital to ensure that it does not leave indelible scars on the children's minds; instead, we need to instill them with resilience, coping mechanisms, and the essential support network which will hold them in good stead over the long run. You may save a life; you never know.

* * * *

Case study: Adolescent Girl (Anonymous)

A young fourteen-year-old girl with severe depression, suicidality, chronic headaches, PTSD, post-concussion syndrome, and neuropathic leg pain resulting from a traumatic fall failed multiple antidepressant and analgesic modalities and presented to a hospital with suicidal ideation. While in the hospital, all of her exams and tests came back normal. She had spent two months in the hospital previously for depression and suicidality, having attempted suicide multiple times in the past with a shoestring and pillow cover. She tried just about every medication available to ease her leg pain: non-steroidal anti-inflammatory agents, acetaminophen, antidepressants, gabapentinoids, anti-seizure medications, and opioid medications. She even had CBT and epidural steroid injections. The doctors tried everything to control this child's pain without success. During this hospital admission, they gave her an intravenous ketamine infusion for one week. On day one, her pain numerical rating scale (NRS) was 7/10. After being on a ketamine infusion for 24 hours, her pain NRS score was a little lower at 5/10. Her mood improved significantly, and she had no further suicidal ideation. On day three, the child's pain NRS score was still 5/10, and on day four, it was 4/10. She had functional movement in her leg because the pain was decreased. On day five, her pain NRS score was a 0/10 and her mood was markedly improved. For the first time, she could take part in physical therapy without pain. Her psychiatric reassessment determined her to be no longer at suicide risk, and she was released from the hospital with follow-up to her outpatient psychiatrist. Her relief lasted for nearly six months until she was readmitted because of a suicide attempt. She was again given an intravenous ketamine infusion, and she experienced the same relief as before.[60]

CHAPTER FIVE

US Veterans, First Responders, Suicide, and Ketamine

"The mind of another is like a black forest."

—*old Russian proverb*

Suicide is a permanent solution to a temporary problem. Every day we see quotes such as "Good News: Combat is no longer the leading killer of soldiers. Bad News: Suicide is now the leading killer," or "The war on veteran suicide starts at home," or "I am basically left with nothing. Too trapped in a war to be at peace, too damaged to be at war."

Suicide rates among veterans and active military personnel are sobering; it has been increasing for the past twenty years and is chronically underrecognized. The rate has been increasing among veterans ages 18 to 34 since 2005, according to the Costs of War study.[1] Veteran suicide occurs at nearly double the general population's rate; current Veteran Affairs (VA) statistics cite that around twenty service members and veterans are lost to suicide every day, or 6,000 per year; however, even this may be a gross underestimate. In September 2022, a new study published by America's Warrior Partnership, Duke University, and the University of Alabama indicated the number of veterans' suicides could be forty-four suicides per day; this number is much higher than current VA records show.[2] It could even be worse because the study counted suicides from 2014 to 2018 and only went up to 64 years old.

Military suicides date back to ancient times. Governments are in the business of training professional soldiers to use physical force to defend their society against the enemy. The inherent risk of injury and death from war exposes veterans to severe physical and mental trauma. The military prepares service members for participation in violence and the rigors of military life with protective resources while also making it easier, more accessible, and even intuitive for them to cause harm. Soldiers use weapons to kill others and themselves, and the reasons veterans commit suicide are not very different from those of anyone else; the main difference is perhaps that the actions leading up to suicide go unnoticed.

Veterans own more guns than others and thus most often use a firearm to commit suicide. In fact, owning a gun triples the risk of dying by suicide.[3] Many soldiers return home from a tour of duty, where they have faced violent combat experiences, only to find themselves isolated and alone. Most veterans who die by suicide do so within a year of leaving the military. About 25 percent of all suicide attempts occur within five minutes of the decision to commit suicide, and three-quarters of veterans who successfully ended their lives had received no form of health care from the VA. The loss of over 60,000 veterans to suicide over the last decade is a bleak statistic.

Governments rarely hesitate to spend money to send soldiers to war, but they falter in paying for the problems soldiers encounter upon returning home. Thousands of soldiers experience difficulties getting appropriate mental-health care within the VA hospital system, resulting in delays in treatment, and many die by suicide while waiting for care. The VA has a history of setbacks and missteps. In 2015, Hillary Clinton was famously quoted saying that many surveys show that veterans were satisfied with VA medical care.[4] This is not the sentiment of most veterans. In fairness, much like socialized medicine, the VA provides excellent care for emergencies such as heart attacks or dealing with cancer. Nevertheless, a problem emerges when confronting mental-health care concerns.

Reducing veteran suicide is a top priority for the VA, but the efforts are failing. Every presidential administration since WWII has "rolled out" strategies to reduce veteran suicide, directing millions of dollars into various programs and calling it a national security crisis. In 2019, then-President Trump rolled out an executive order known as the President's Road Map to Empower Veterans and End a National Tragedy of Suicide (PREVENTS), which was billed as eleven different governmental departments and private firms forming a task force to create a strategy to study the factors contributing to veteran suicide.[5, 6] The task force recommended funding suicide prevention programs at the federal level; however, the pandemic delayed the task force. The initiative aimed to increase awareness that suicide is both preventable and treatable by encouraging employers and academic institutions to provide mental health and wellness practices and increase suicide-prevention training.

The military has taken steps to become proactive toward suicide prevention through screening for psychological disorders called Comprehensive Soldier Fitness. This screening tool represents the army's decision to place an equal emphasis on psychological and physical strength.[7] Younger soldiers are being recruited nowadays, and many present with preexisting psychological disorders. Basic training, sleep deprivation, loss of family support, foreign environment, combat, and anxiety about deployment all increase the stressors related to the military. Still, it is important to remember having a mental disorder alone does not predict suicidal behavior, and equally, many soldiers who end their lives by suicide had no history of mental health issues. Military screening efforts to determine risk incorporate exercises to evaluate a person's distress in response to adverse situations, such as hand-to-hand combat. Also, the ability to problem solve, seek help through adaptive methods, and assess the likelihood of acting on impulses to escape undesirable situations are methods employed by the military. Resilience training is a line of defense against suicide, as it helps with coping skills and reducing self-blame. Despite these forward steps, genuine progress in suicide among veterans is still out of reach.

Post-traumatic stress disorder (PTSD), sometimes referred to as shell shock or combat stress, was made famous by the 1978 movie *The Deer*

Hunter starring Robert De Niro and Christopher Walken. Traumatic military experiences can bring about PTSD and contribute to suicide. As many as 13 percent of combat veterans have PTSD, which is undoubtedly an underestimate since many veterans have a stigma against mental health and hide their emotions.[8] Combat exposure, injury, grief, hostile unit climate, and family-related stressors, as well as physical, sexual, financial, and acute health problems, are all too familiar but often unnoticed stress-related circumstances among soldiers. Combat exposure causes significant prolonged stress, requiring many of those deployed to be on constant guard from any unfriendly fire, improvised explosive devices (IEDs), and other dangers while patrolling civilian areas. The prolonged and repeated nature of deployments and the uncertainty about whether one's tour will be extended create a significant burden on soldiers and their families. These factors increase the likelihood of PTSD, which has a significant association with suicidal behavior. In 2018, the US Department of Veterans Affairs spent 17 billion dollars on disability payments for over one million veterans with PTSD. Approximately half to one-third of people do not find relief through treatment, and PTSD can become a lifelong, chronic, and debilitating disease.

Combat survivors with severe injuries and PTSD are at higher risk of taking their lives by suicide. Medical advances have created new life-saving interventions extending survival in the face of severe injuries. Paradoxically, those who survive horrific injuries are stranded and left alone to deal with serious health problems, including disabilities and disfigurements. Traumatic brain injury (TBI) is a particular flag for suicide risk among military populations. Seldom discussed is the fact that there is a high prevalence of TBI among military personnel because of the widespread exposure to IEDs and blast injuries resulting in head trauma.[9] The 2009 movie *The Hurt Locker* highlighted the realities of soldiers exposed to IEDs and TBIs. Traumatic brain injury increases the risk of depression and PTSD, and the neuro-psychological consequences of TBI are aggression, disinhibition, and impulsivity. Combine all these elements with a firearm, and the likelihood of successful suicide is better than 99 percent.

Military tribalism is another poorly discussed topic. Soldiers in combat often exhibit a strong tribal mentality. Soldiers are entrusted with protecting each other in extremely difficult situations. Some of the strongest human bonds are forged during combat. Humans, as primates, desire to belong and long for connection. Military soldiers in combat will sacrifice, kill, and die for their group. Once a soldier leaves the group environment, a sense of losing one's identity can contribute to mental illness.

People afflicted with PTSD are associated with an increased risk of depression and suicide. PTSD is the technical name for a complex of problems that arise in the wake of a trauma. Symptoms of PTSD fall into three categories:

- Re-experiencing (e.g., nightmares)
- Avoidance (e.g., avoid talking about the event)
- Arousal (e.g., difficulty sleeping)

Service members with PTSD likely perpetrated, witnessed, or experienced the horrors of war, causing an overwhelming sense of fear, which triggers an alarm system within the amygdala and other areas of the brain.[10] PTSD is akin to a well-rehearsed traumatic memory that repeats in a complex network of nerves in the brain through the Default Mode Network (DMN). Every time that memory is activated, it strengthens the DMN for those memories.[11] Memories are repeatedly brought up through specific noises, songs, events, words, smells, or other sensations. Then the narrative becomes integrated into life like a bad habit, impacting one's life. This renders the individual incapable of turning off the biological fight-or-flight response to the "danger." PTSD is an actual physiological and psychological response to traumatic events. When false alarms trigger a PTSD reaction, the body automatically perceives the stress and reacts. The diagnosis of PTSD requires symptoms lasting for about one month and resulting in distress and impairment in social functioning. Veterans describe flashbacks, memory loss, fear, and startle reactions, all closely associated with mental illness and suicidal behaviors. Often the victims suppress or hide the memories of their experiences, resulting in mental and physical health problems later in life. Carrying the diagnosis of a mental health disorder decreases a person's life span significantly.[12] Furthermore, the intense stress from PTSD is associated with an increased risk of heart disease in a brief period,[13] and another study showed altered brain tissue.[14]

The Treatment of PTSD

Treating veterans with PTSD is complex, and the poor prognosis and public health burden of PTSD necessitate the development of more effective and broader treatment approaches. There are many facets to successfully treating PTSD. We will be focusing on psychedelics and cognitive therapy in this chapter.

Psychedelics help PTSD by providing relief to the mind, body, and spirit. This can be broken down into psychological trauma, addiction, physiological benefits, and spiritual connections. Psychedelics assist the mind in getting out of the ingrained traumatic memories that perpetrate the mind through the DMN. This concept will be expanded more in a later chapter.

Psychedelics like ketamine, MDMA, ibogaine, DMT, and psilocybin are showing promising results in veterans with PTSD. Yet few politicians want to hear about paying for psychedelics for veterans. Ironically, psychedelics were outlawed by Presidents Johnson and Nixon because of concerns that they were fueling opposition to the Vietnam War and other government activities. Only now, after a sixty-year hiatus, are we reconsidering these valuable medications for mental illness. New studies are underway treating veterans with psychedelics.[15] Stanford University has been using the psychedelic ibogaine and fMRI to treat veterans with PTSD; they have reported improvements in cognitive functioning and creating new neural pathways (neuroplasticity). Portland and San Diego are conducting trials with psilocybin and MDMA.

Considering the crippling psychological weight of these factors, we return our focus to the importance of ketamine. Many studies have evaluated the safety and efficacy of repeated doses of ketamine and other psychedelics to reduce PTSD symptoms in both active military personnel and veterans.[16, 17] The idea of using ketamine for treating PTSD comes from the wars in Afghanistan and Iraq. The military routinely uses ketamine for soldiers during surgery and treatment of burns sustained in Afghanistan and Iraq. Ketamine had the unexpected benefit of reducing the incidence of PTSD by 50 percent compared to those who were treated with other anesthetics.[18] The army even did a study to ensure ketamine did not worsen PTSD and concluded that it indeed helped PTSD.[19] In 2014, Adriana Feder studied forty-one soldiers with chronic PTSD and treated them with ketamine; nearly three-quarters of them improved their depression and PTSD symptom severity. The improvements persisted, and side effects, such as feelings of dissociation, were mild and transient.

Psychedelics and PTSD became a popular topic with the "Trauma Interventions using Mindfulness-Based Extinction and Reconsolidation" (TIMBER) study. Researchers combined mindfulness psychotherapy and ketamine to treat PTSD.[20] They found TIMBER's introductory rationale was grounded in the healing, mindfulness, and resiliency-building properties of yoga.[21] Treatment resulted in the remission of PTSD symptoms and perceptible improvements in depression, panic symptoms, insomnia, and attentiveness. In interviews with Dr. Basant Pradhan, he discussed that TIMBER has also been found efficacious for clients with addiction to alcohol, opioids, and nicotine.

Veterans who have undergone treatment with psychedelics have varied experiences. Dr. John Krystal published a paper on a group of soldiers with PTSD.[22] After treating them with ketamine infusions, they found that their depression was effectively better than after a placebo. Still, the study failed to find a significant dose-related effect of ketamine on PTSD symptoms. However, Dr. Krystal suggested in a podcast with Tim Ferriss that it is important to do therapy prior to ketamine sessions to better treat PTSD symptoms, and this may account for the result. Even more, having an experienced military psychotherapist who is also a veteran can have an even more beneficial result. Undoubtedly, these veterans are leaning into the hardest work of their lives as they come face to face with things they may have been avoiding—sometimes for decades—since their deployment.

Independent of which psychedelic was used, many report the first experience to be very intense. A 2012 study questioned seventy-two veterans who attempted suicide, and every one of them spoke about their desire to end the intense emotional distress created by the treatment.[23] Combat veterans describe the treatment bringing up blood and gore memories from the war, or nightmare-like hallucinations of trying desperately to pull the trigger, the magazine falling out, or the barrel melting. With subsequent treatments, the experiences become less intense. The psychedelic experience can lead to closure for some veterans. For example, a soldier might describe being in a dreamlike state, and the fallen soldiers from his unit would approach, dressed in white, and place their hands on his shoulder and say, "Hey man, it's OK, I am in a good place." Psychedelics can help unlock subconscious traumas and allow the person to confront them. Often, there are other traumas from childhood that have never been addressed. After the experience, many describe that a heavy weight has been lifted and that life improves.

****

Case Study: Navy Seal and Afghanistan Veteran (Anonymous)

My ketamine treatment was unlike anything I'd ever experienced before. I'm still processing it and trying to quantify the benefits. First, the facility was first-class and conducive to a very positive experience. The treatment room was modern and comfortable. I was briefed on the procedure and given assurances that the treatment was safe and controlled. At the start of the treatment, I felt very peaceful and lighthearted. Having a board-certified anesthesiologist and my family in the room gave me added assurance, which became increasingly meaningful as the treatment progressed. I closed my eyes and tried to relax and enjoy the tranquility. I quickly drifted off and was taken into what seemed to be another dimension. It felt like I was traveling upwards, often without a sense of gravity or time, and my surroundings were constantly changing as if walls were folding in on themselves. As I continued deeper into these dimensions, I wondered at times how I would return. That's when knowing a trusted family member was present became important. Even though I had seemingly lost touch with reality, I knew someone was there to bring me back eventually. At several points during the experience, I thought I was fully awake and back in the treatment room, only to find myself drifting off into another dream world. As I began to come back to reality, I continued to drift in and out of the dream world, but I was relieved to come back to the real world finally. I felt a sense of relief and happiness knowing I was safely back home with my family members who were waiting for me in the treatment room. As I continue to process the experience, the primary takeaway was the sense of happiness that I was back home with my family and in control of my life. This may have a very beneficial therapeutic effect for those who have lost an appreciation for the things we often take for granted, like family, being alive, and having control of your life.[24]

****

Healthcare Professional Suicide

Unbeknownst to many, the US has a September National Physician Suicide Awareness Day (#NPSADay). More than half of physicians know a physician or colleague who has either considered, attempted, or died by suicide in their career. Despite often being considered heroes, healthcare workers are vulnerable to post-traumatic stress the same as anyone else. Healthcare workers are dying of suicide at surprising rates. Historically, physicians have one of the highest suicide rates of any profession, at about 300 per year in the United States.[25] In particular, emergency room physicians are at high risk.

To understand why doctors would want to end their lives by suicide, a closer look at the journey through medical school is helpful. In medical school, there is a strong sense of community even while competing fiercely against one another for the top grades in the class. Medical students are typically shielded against social isolation because they are all doing the same seemingly impossible job, constantly learning and trying to become the best doctors possible. The medical school becomes the tribe. When you are in the tribe, making friends is easy. But when graduation happens, students are sent out to face the medical field alone, and making friends and having social support becomes more difficult. It is akin to being in war together and suddenly the fight is over and the tribe separates. This is what medical school is like for just about everyone. All the people you became very close to and depended on for social support, study support, and emotional support suddenly disappear and you may never see them again. It is an emotional roller coaster that takes a lot of time to figure out. Then in private practice, we all become incredibly busy trying to handle our new lives in the clinic, hospital, family, and new environments. It is no wonder many medical doctors become depressed after medical school. Most of us know to blow off stress in a healthy way, but some fall into severe depression and ultimately take their own lives.

Doctors and nurses exist in a profession that encourages "toughing it out" and "not complaining." Many barriers exist in healthcare that prohibit a culture of well-being, as physicians and nurses "stuff" their feelings in a bag at the workplace. For example, during medical rotations, medical students and residents often endure a lot of mental and verbal abuse, primarily due to the hierarchy that exists among physicians. This is challenging because when patients' lives are on the line, feelings and respect are often thrown out the door.

One physician has dedicated her life's work to preventing physician suicide. Pamela Wible, MD, is America's leading voice on medical care and doctor suicide. She has operated a free doctor suicide helpline since 2012. She says "physician burnout" is a misnomer—a harmful term that distracts from the human rights violations doctors experience in training and practice. Physicians are not Navy SEALS and should not be trained like frontline special forces. Dr. Wible feels that medical schools and residency programs must address hazardous working conditions that lead to lifelong mental and physical health conditions in our physicians. She further explains that nobody knows the true physician suicide rate since the data is concealed due to stigma. For example, physician anesthesiologist suicides often occur as overdoses and are listed as "accidents" on the death certificate. She thinks we lose more than 400 doctors each year in the US, and this is not including medical student suicides.

The touching story of Dr. Lorna Breen, the director of a Manhattan hospital emergency department, is especially relevant:[26]

Dr. Breen's hospital was overwhelmed with an influx of COVID-19 patients. Returning from vacation, she was confronted with issues like inadequate personal protective equipment and lack of ventilators. Shortly after, she tested positive for COVID-19 and self-quarantined at home to recover.

In a period of three weeks, Dr. Breen had treated patients with COVID-19, contracted the virus herself, recovered, and returned to work.

On April 1st, her first day back on the job, she faced a colossal workload; she and her colleagues were working 24/7, with patients dying in the hallways and experiencing post-COVID symptoms from which she herself was still suffering. She and her colleagues worked with limited protection, few hospital beds, and a lack of resources. She was simultaneously covering two hospitals five miles from each other. It was as bad as everyone had heard—there were intubated patients on stretchers jammed in the hallways, a shortage of oxygen tanks, and the radiology department was serving as a hospice center for patients dying from COVID-19. It was a seemingly impossible situation. Dr. Breen knew she could not help patients how she wanted, and quitting was not an option. During the pandemic's peak, nearly a quarter of all people admitted to the emergency department with COVID-19 would die.

On April 9, 2020, sounding unlike herself, Dr. Breen called her sister from her Manhattan apartment, reporting that she could not even get up from a chair. She was nearly catatonic and was uttering only two-word sentences, if you could even call them that. A chain of friends and family drove her to Charlottesville, Virginia, where she was admitted to a psychiatric ward for eleven days.

On April 21, Dr. Breen left the hospital. Things seemed better, and she started going out for long runs. However, five days later, she took her own life. She died of self-inflicted wounds at the University of Virginia Hospital.

The tragic case of Dr. Breen is interesting because she had no prior history of mental illness, depression, or anxiety. Intelligent and motivated, her commitment and drive were impressive. She was enrolled in the Cornell executive MBA/MS health care leadership degree. Most of us do not think we will be gone from this earth by age forty-nine. To better understand her suicide and why the COVID-19 crisis played such a crucial role, it is essential to consider Dr. Breen's life before the COVID-19 crisis.

Lorna Breen's father was a doctor and her mom a nurse. Yearning to become a doctor from an early age, she graduated from the Wyoming Seminary class in 1988. Dr. Breen was a consummate overachiever, graduating from medical school and completing two residencies—internal and emergency medicine. She spent as much time in residency as many neurosurgeons—eighteen years of education after high school.

She was an avid snowboarder and marathon runner who enjoyed playing cello in an orchestra and salsa dancing. Dr. Breen had to put her life on hold when COVID-19 hit. The stress, insomnia, and anxiety took their toll on her. She spent a week and a half at home to recover from COVID and then insisted on returning to work, but something changed. Her family notes, "Something about her was not there." Although she had no apparent history of severe depression, it's arguable Dr. Breen displayed symptoms after the COVID-19 infection. Her father, a well-respected trauma surgeon, explained in a television interview that she was not the same after the infection.

So what was it, after the COVID-19 infection, that caused her to have a mental breakdown requiring admission to a psychiatric institution? Perhaps if the culture were different, doctors could reveal when they are suffering from mental illness instead of repressing, ignoring, or hiding their symptoms. Dr. Breen was fearful that she would lose her medical license or be ostracized at work if she acknowledged that she needed help. Doctors are comfortable diagnosing and treating trauma but are reluctant to reveal their own mental health issues for fear of ruining their careers.

Healthcare workers were struggling to cope and facing unprecedented challenges:

- Inadequate personal protective equipment
- Exposure to family members
- Sick colleagues
- Overwhelmed facilities
- Fear of medical board punishment
- Work stress

Finally, consider that even medical professionals who are familiar with mental-health resources seldom ask for help. Imagine the impact upon people who don't know about the resources, recognize the warning signs, or get help. Dr. Breen's family has set up a foundation to raise awareness about physician burnout and to safeguard their well-being (https://drlornabreen. org/).

First Responder Suicides

After a routine shift, twenty-eight-year-old Richland County sheriff Derek Fish returned to his cruiser and shot himself with his service revolver. In response to this incident, Leon Lott, a fellow Richland County sheriff, expressed the dire need for a change in how law enforcement addresses suicide and mental health problems.[27]

First responder (police officers, firefighters, etc.) suicide statistics are vague as no federal agency officially counts the number of suicides in the law-enforcement community. The National Police Suicide Foundation (NPS) has attempted to document police suicides; they also provide suicide awareness and prevention training programs.[28]

A recent study found that police officers and firefighters are far more likely to die by suicide than in the line of duty.[29] According to the study, there were at least 103 firefighter suicides and 140 police officer suicides in one year (2019). In contrast, 93 firefighters and 129 police officers died in the line of duty. In 2020, at least 228 police officers died by suicide, whereas 132 officers died in the line of duty; this is a 25 percent increase from 2019. Mainstream media outlets seldom cover first responder suicides, and the public remains largely unaware of the issue. A 2021 movie called *The Guilty* is about the mental health of first responders and attempts to highlight the issues normally not spoken about, but that are prevalent everywhere.

First-responder suicides are not considered "line-of-duty deaths," and surviving families often receive no financial compensation. Approximately 90 percent of police officers who commit suicide in the US do so with a firearm. Limiting access to these weapons is not feasible when considering an officer's need for them in the field. Most suicides are traced to depression and PTSD, which stem from constant exposure to death and violence.

As a society, we must open the discussion about mental illness among the first responder community, including firefighters and police officers. Suicide is the most catastrophic of consequences for failing to treat mental illness. First responders often experience PTSD and depression but feel pressured to hide mental health challenges because of the cultural stigma. In police departments, an omerta or code of secrecy exists around mental illness. The topic is uneasy to talk about or approach. One officer reported, "When I was involved in my first shooting, I was cleared right away, and I was not given any administrative time off. Basically, they bought you a beer and told you that you were a hero. I had to deal with it all on my own, and there were no department resources or even a chaplain."

It is surprising and shocking that more officers die by their own hands than by other causes. More officers have died of suicide than in shootings and traffic accidents combined. Among the 228 police officers who died by suicide in 2020, approximately 25 percent were veterans with at least twenty years of service.[30, 31] Work-related stress and depression are commonplace in police work. It's tough, especially in large cities like New York City or St. Louis. Law enforcement is among the most harrowing career fields in the world. Consider the strain involved in dealing with criminals and victims of accidents, verbal and physical abuse, gang violence, murder, and suicide. The sheer volume of negative memories can be catastrophic.

Some organizations have recommended police officers receive some mental health care annually from a therapist versed in dealing with first responder stress and trauma. In Idaho, a crisis line specific to first responders has opened for use. The Albemarle County Department of Fire and Rescue in Virginia is providing mental health resources for firefighters who deal with trauma from helping others.

One officer with twenty-four years of police service describes how he found himself alone in his bedroom with his gun drawn and ready to shoot himself. Luckily, his wife walked in and kept him from going through with the suicide. Psychologists diagnosed him with PTSD and depression, and he started both therapy and medication.

The January 6 Capitol riot was a stark reminder of a country divided. Few realize that four Washington, DC[32] officers committed suicide shortly after the riot. These officers had over fifty years of service between them.

Here is the experience of one officer who took his life shortly after the riots:

On January 6, at 2:38 p.m., Officer Jeffrey Smith sent his wife a text, "London has fallen." This was in response to the start of the Capitol riot and a reference to a movie about a plan to assassinate world leaders attending a funeral in Britain. Along with 850 other DC police officers, Smith was at the Capitol on January 6 where over seventy officers were injured. Around 5:35 p.m., he was in the Capitol building fighting the rioters when they hurled a metal pole that struck his helmet and face shield. He continued working into the night. At 9:00 p.m., he told two supervisors he was in pain from being hit by the pole and later visited the police medical clinic at 10:15 p.m. On his police injury form, he wrote: "Hit with a flying object in face shield and helmet" and "Began feeling pain in my neck and face." He left the clinic at 1:31 a.m., was placed on sick leave, and was sent home with pain medications. According to his wife in a *Washington Post* interview, Smith seemed in constant pain and was unable to turn his head. He did not leave the house or go outside to walk their dog as he had usually done. He refused to talk to other people or watch television and spoke little about the riots. His wife described him in the days that followed as dealing with insomnia, waking during the night, and pacing about. Mrs. Smith says, "He was not the same Jeff that left on the sixth. . . . " On January 14, Smith returned to the police clinic for a follow-up appointment and was ordered back to work. The next afternoon, he left the house for an overnight shift, taking the ham-and-turkey sandwiches his wife had packed. On his way to the District, Smith used his firearm to shoot himself in the head.[33, 34]

CHAPTER SIX

Addiction, Suicide, and Psychedelics

"It's a big club, and we're all in it."

—*George Carlin*

Drug Overdoses and Addiction

Edgar Allan Poe once wrote, "I have no pleasure in the stimulants in which I sometimes so madly indulge. It has not been in the pursuit of pleasure that I have periled life and reputation and reason. It has been in the desperate attempt to escape torturing memories . . ." Addiction does not develop overnight, is certainly nothing new, and affects all walks of life. At first, recreational drugs may seem almost magical. But gradually, the drugs start to make decisions—eventually the most crucial life decisions—for you, taking away your freedom and autonomy.

Certainly, the manner in which people use the word addiction in everyday language is diverse. Four hundred years ago, addiction implied a devoted or habitual behavior in a religious sense. In contrast, today, it is framed as a disease involving central nervous system imbalances. Most define addiction as a behavioral pattern in which the person's choices lead to a loss of control. A person can be addicted to just about anything. What is important is to realize that addiction is bonded to our behaviors. There are positive and harmful addictions. For addictive behavior to become harmful, it often must be associated with extreme behaviors that do not cease when a person desires to do so. This is why it is estimated that about 210 million people use addictive substances in the US and about 10 percent become addicted negatively.[1]

Grasping the breadth of addiction is difficult. Visualize the Vietnam War Memorial wall in Washington DC. Now, imagine that same wall for all those Americans who died from drug overdoses in the same period. That wall would measure over one mile. Yet, there's no outrage for these unfortunate people who have died, unlike that from the Vietnam War. According to CDC data, 20 million people in the United States are addicted to a substance.[2] Those numbers are rising. Some states have been hit particularly hard by the drug overdose crisis due to the seemingly uncontrollable amounts of fentanyl flooding across the US-Mexico border. In 2022, Montana law enforcement seized fifty-eight times more fentanyl in six months than was seized in all of 2019.[3]

Internationally, Iceland and Sweden score very high in every ranking of quality of life and social equity, yet the number of drug-related deaths in these countries is sky-high. The National Institute for Health and Welfare has shown that overdose deaths by fentanyl are up in Iceland, overdose deaths by heroin are up in Sweden, and overdose deaths from buprenorphine have increased in Finland.[4]

The overdose problem is a public health crisis costing thousands of lives, with opioids and lockdowns driving the numbers up. In 2021, a total of 107,622 Americans died of drug overdoses, the most ever recorded. That is a death every five minutes around the clock. Compare this to 91,000 in 2020 or 70,000 in 2018. About 379 million deadly doses of fentanyl were seized in 2022 by Drug Enforcement Administration (DEA), enough to kill every American.[5]

Addiction experts blame the pandemic for leaving people isolated and disrupting treatment and vital recovery programs. In addition, there's a lack of mental health providers and a more robust drug supply. Many emergency rooms are experiencing thousand-percent increases in overdose cases.[6, 7] These problems are not exclusive to adults; drug overdoses affect children. A study from the journal *Pediatrics* showed a rise in child drug overdoses during the pandemic.

New York, Seattle, San Francisco, Las Vegas, and other cities report an increase in overdose deaths.[8] Daniel Buccino, the John Hopkins Broadway Center for Addiction clinical manager, says, "We are seeing more of those cases going straight to the morgue rather than to the emergency department." Ninety-three thousand people died from drug overdoses in 2020 and 107,622 in 2022; over 70 percent were from fentanyl. In drug addiction hot spots like San Francisco, overdose deaths increased by 173 percent between 2018 and 2020, with over 800 drug overdoses in 2020 compared to 254 deaths from COVID-19. Opioid overdose deaths in San Francisco would be far worse if not for the over 4,300 times the drug Narcan (naltrexone) was administered; Narcan reverses opioids and is akin to a fire extinguisher for opioid overdoses. More alarming, the Narcan data from the Drug Overdose Prevention project is self-reported and is probably a major undercount.

One reason for the deepening of the opioid crisis is the rapid increase in fentanyl, which is fifty times more powerful than heroin or morphine. Fentanyl remains in the body longer than heroin, overpowers the respiratory system, and causes people to stop breathing. The brain habituates and becomes comfortable with a lack of oxygen called hypoxia. It may not happen the first time, but eventually, it goes horribly wrong and death ensues. Even more disturbing is that children two and three years old are dying from ingesting fentanyl. According to federal mortality data, there were over 133 opioid-related deaths among children younger than three in 2021.[9]

Most overdose deaths occur in low-income apartment buildings and city-funded homeless shelters; many others have died needlessly on sidewalks and parks. In Oregon, drugs have been decriminalized, but the overdose death rate has only risen, mainly due to an influx of fentanyl and methamphetamines.[10] Oregon's drug problem is only getting worse despite over $300 million spent on services for addicted individuals; this is also in part due to a rapidly changing drug supply, lack of law enforcement, and shortage of mental health services.

This is not the world's first opioid crisis. In the 1700s, Great Britain flooded China with opium, derailing its economy and population. Today, China manufactures fentanyl, which flows over the US-Mexico border, and the Mexican cartels are all too happy to manufacture and facilitate its US distribution. On the "business" side of illegal drugs, according to the DEA, the pandemic also disrupted the supply of drugs from Mexico, which heightened risks for users who sought new dealers and bought unfamiliar products. These unforeseen and dangerous consequences resulted in a rash of overdoses and deaths. People with a history of substance abuse experience higher levels of psychological stress, and these behaviors may persist for years after a pandemic has ended.

Why are so many people falling into substance abuse and addiction? The American Society of Addiction Medicine (ASAM) defines addiction as a treatable, chronic medical disease involving complex interactions among brain circuits, genetics, the environment, and an individual's life experiences. Addiction, at its core, is the repetition of traumatic, ingrained memories. For example, every time you activate the memory and use alcohol, you enjoy the feeling, and that memory strengthens. The trauma memories are repeatedly rehearsed until they become entrenched in the Default Mode Network (DMN). Each time you use alcohol, or any substance, for that matter, you like the feeling a little more, and then you begin to use it more frequently. The alcohol-related memories have more power over how you think and act; before long, alcohol makes your most crucial life decisions.

Prolonged isolation is the worst thing for drug addicts. The pandemic left many isolated in their homes, exacerbating feelings of uncertainty, insecurity, and hopelessness. Lockdowns reduced contact between people by as much as 75 percent, and thousands relapsed into substance abuse, exposing them to the high risk of death from overdose.[11] The Rat Park theory of drug dependency demonstrates the disastrous consequences of isolation.[12] Dr. Bruce Alexander showed that when rats are isolated, they drink the drugged water and overdose 100 percent of the time. When the rats were happy and bonded in their environment, they avoided the drugged water. Humans react much in the same way as Dr. Alexander's rats. When we are homeless, we use drugs nearly 100 percent of the time, and when we live in stable family environments, we usually avoid them. Relapse rates for substance abuse disorders are high, ranging between 40 and 80 percent, even with traditional treatment. A forty-eight-year-old West Virginia man, just being alone for five days, became anxious and depressed and relapsed into taking his opioid painkiller. His original addiction followed shoulder surgery. He blames his relapse on the isolation and loneliness from the lockdowns. Once he was called back to work, he stopped the drugs.[13]

Hungarian-born Canadian physician Gabor Maté is a bestselling author sought after for his expertise on trauma, addiction, stress, and childhood development. He has worked with countless addicts and dealt with his own addictions. His book *The Myth of Normal* recounts the many reasons people become addicted.[14] One major reason is the trauma people have endured. Maté posits that addiction is not simply a disease or because of bad choices or genes. The studies claiming that genetics causes our addictions are highly flawed.[15] Despite the millions of dollars and years of psychiatric research, no one has ever identified any genes that cause mental illness or any group of genes that code for specific mental health conditions or are required for the presence of mental disorders. No single addiction gene has ever been found or ever will be. A predisposition to a disease is not the same as a predetermination. As with any behavioral trait, it is likely that many genes are involved in the development of addiction, but there is certainly more to the story.

The environment turns genes on and off. We understand this from cancer and nutrition research. Any risk of genetic involvement for addiction can be reliably offset by being raised in a loving, stable, nurturing environment. Addiction is not someone drawing a short genetic straw; it is more about the environment and coping mechanisms. Twin and adoption studies prove little if anything. Psychologist Jay Joseph criticizes twin studies that compare identical twins and same-sex fraternal twin pairs in the same family home. Few studies research what are called "reared-apart" twins. Joseph shows the many methodological flaws of twin studies based on outright false assumptions. Even more, it is important to remember that what is considered addiction in one culture is not necessarily considered addiction in another. For example, daily marijuana use in Jamaica is not looked upon negatively, as it is in the United States.

Most people's pain and traumas happen very early on. For kids who are exposed to suicide, the event becomes a consequential, life-defining trauma, just like it did for me and for Gavin de Becker. A child's closeness with parents or guardians who have adequate emotional availability promotes healthy brain development, but the lack of it impedes healthy development. The culmination of our personal and social life events shapes our brains. Most people experiencing addiction have a history of trauma, often starting in infancy.

An addiction serves as an escape from torturing memories. We must look closely at people's life experiences to understand what they really need in order to avoid or break the cycle of addiction. Addiction takes on physical symptoms and cycles of remission and relapse, tissue damage, and even death. Addiction could be seen as a natural response to terrible circumstances and an attempt to soothe pain incurred in childhood and stresses in adulthood.

Most concepts of mental health and addiction see the brain separate from the body, but treating addiction must include mind, body, and spirit. Although a more extensive discussion, one must wonder how we arrived at this biological-mental disease paradigm. While mental ailments seem to function like diseased organs, mainstream psychiatry attempts to reduce them to DNA-dictated brain chemicals. Alcoholics Anonymous (AA) talks about alcoholism as a disease. AA's language is a big reason why we believe addiction is a disease that can only be treated.[16] In modern medical times, mental illness focuses on medical treatment as the mainstay of therapy. Psychiatry commits the same error as other medical specialties through reductionist thinking, trying to solve complex problems with simple solutions that do not work. For example, it is ridiculous to assume depression in every patient is due to an inherited neurotransmitter deficiency when it's clear that environment, life circumstances, and even diet are all known causes of depression. Yet, the primary treatment for depression is replacing brain neurotransmitters with medications like Prozac. This line of thinking has been around for more than a half a century. We will see how ketamine can be one vital piece in a holistic treatment plan in the next chapter.

Even today, there are no biological laboratory markers measuring mental illness. Certainly, we have research around measuring proteins like BDNF and mTOR in suicide victims, but these are done only in universities. There are no measurable physical markers of mental illness other than the subjective description (mood) and the behaviors (appetite, sleep, self-harm).

On *The Joe Rogan Experience*, Dr. Maté answered the question: why do people get hooked on opiates? It is partially because we are born with an internal opioid system called endorphins. Endorphin molecules are neuropeptides that are produced in the brain and have morphine-like properties. They deliver pain relief, a sense of well-being, and euphoria, similar to other opioids. Endorphins are involved in natural reward circuits, such as exercise, drinking, eating, intimacy, and maternal behaviors. More importantly, they are stimulated each time your mom hugs you. A child who experiences inadequate development of the endorphin brain circuits from lack of maternal stimulation becomes an adult at high risk of opioid addiction.[17] We can show this in the laboratory using infant mice with genetically knocked-out morphine receptors; they stop crying for their mothers when separated. For an animal in the wild, this means certain death. That's how vital endorphins are to animal physiology.

Repeated opioid use causes tolerance to most drugs, including heroin and cocaine. Heroin causes the downregulation of endorphins, opioid receptors, and the production of anti-opioid peptides. Addicts then require increasing amounts of opioids to induce the same level of analgesia, a process known as tolerance. Addiction is a loss of control over drug taking or compulsive drug seeking, despite harmful consequences.

Many heroin users describe using heroin as being like a "warm, soft hug." Another addict said that using helped him to feel normal for the first time in his life. Most of us would think, how can this be? This highlights the importance of parents providing love and nurture to their children with touch as favorable reinforcement. People who cut ("cutters") are not trying to end their lives; instead, they are looking for the release of endorphins, akin to a morphine hit, to relieve both physical and emotional pain.[18]

Dr. Maté was the supervising physician for a drug injection site in one of North America's most concentrated areas of drug abuse in Vancouver, British Columbia. He eloquently describes a story that shows the face of heroin addiction. One of his patients, in for detox, was a large, muscular man, measuring about six feet four, with a shaved head, earrings, and plenty of tattoos. He was asked, what does heroin do for you? He answered in a low voice, "Doc, I don't know how to tell you this exactly. It's like when you are three years old, but imagine you are sick, you have a high fever, you have the chills and shaking all over, and your mother wraps you in a warm blanket, puts you on her lap, and gives you warm chicken soup. That is what heroin feels like." Many famous heroin addicts, such as Russell Brand, Dave Navarro, and Keith Richards, have described similar stories. Dave Navarro said that his heroin addiction gave him a sense of love and acceptance. Interestingly, ketamine plus psychotherapy can result in heroin abstinence and decrease heroin cravings. Some patients were heroin-free even two years after the intervention.[19]

Trauma cuts us into little pieces, letting other parts of your body override and not balancing the body as it should. We become perilous creatures when people become cut off from the heart. All substance abuse can be an escape from the confines of oneself and an attempt to find inner peace, calmness, a sense of self-worth, and comfortable normality. Substance abuse calls people when they feel isolated, unworthy, and lack hope and faith. People are desperate to soothe their pain. This pain is central, and only people in pain request anesthesia. The point is to ask why one has pain, not why one has an addiction. Addiction is ultimately an affliction of the mind, body, and spirit.

As a seven-year-old, I vividly remember my mother being beaten by my drunk father during one of their many fights. I don't exactly recall what happened, but I remember my father pushing my mom down to the ground and dragging her by her hair toward the bedroom. My initial reaction was to push my mom's feet so she would feel less pain from being dragged by her hair. I remember her distinctly looking at me and saying, "thank you." I was confident that she knew I was trying to help. Then I heard the fighting and screams. Then I went to bed. After reading this, you might ask, are you addicted to anything? Not exactly. Thankfully, instead of turning to substance abuse while growing up, I took up running. My reaction to running was natural, and I have never stopped running.

Addiction is so much more than a disease because it causes negative consequences, and the person refuses to give it up. Calling addiction a disease does not go far enough and prevents us from moving toward healing. Not all addictions are created equal. In a sense, there are big "T" and small "t" traumas.[20] Addiction depends on the magnitude of the trauma needing soothing as well as the internal relation to the trauma. Most people discount their childhood traumas until something helps uncover them. People find their talking points about their happy childhoods have many blind spots. Addiction is a complex physical, emotional, biological, physiological, and spiritual process. Everything is connected.

Ketamine-Assisted Psychotherapy: How Ketamine Helps Addiction

As mentioned, ketamine is but one step in treating mental health disorders, and we must focus on the connection between mind, body, and spirit. Psychotherapy is a critical component of any psychedelic treatment, and psychotherapy alone is effective in treating depression and suicidal ideation. A study published at Stony Brook University found that even one telehealth session with a counselor can be beneficial. Even after a single meeting, people reported that feelings of anxiety and hopelessness improved. But combining psychotherapy with psychedelic treatment is more effective than therapy alone, as researchers like Phil Wolfson, Lori Calabrese, and Celia Morgan have clearly shown.[21, 22]

The research is clear that medications or psychedelics alone are not as effective as combining it with some type of psychotherapy. Ketamine-assisted psychotherapy uses a dosage escalation strategy to achieve different mental states, ranging from euphoria to full out-of-body experiences. Johns Hopkins University is conducting clinical research with psilocybin-assisted therapy, which is currently in phase 3 FDA trials. Currently, ketamine is the only legally available psychedelic medication for assisted psychotherapy.

Dr. Phil Wolfson is the president of the Ketamine Research Foundation and specializes in ketamine-assisted psychotherapy. The effectiveness of ketamine-assisted psychotherapy depends on several factors. Depending on the dose, ketamine promotes a timeout of sorts from ordinary thoughts, a relief from negative emotions, and an openness to expanding the mind with access to "the self." Patients often report feeling like they are part of the cosmos, experiencing different colors and light, and can feel more connected with their environment in ways not otherwise possible.

These effects enhance the patient's ability to engage in meaningful psychotherapy during and after administration. It is potent for recovery from depression and the lingering effects of trauma. One or two sessions are necessary to find the optimal amount of ketamine for an individual. The sessions can be intensive, fatiguing, and can last for up to three hours, but ketamine-assisted psychotherapy is rewarding for its practitioners and their patients. He and his colleagues have created online sharing groups. Dr. Wolfson attests no one comes back the same after a ketamine treatment.

Dr. Wolfson published a paper on the safety of ketamine where a significant portion of the patients were over sixty-five. He has safely treated many geriatric patients. Dr. Wolfson is seventy-seven and uses ketamine on himself with no untoward effects. His oldest patient is eighty-seven and has done very well with ketamine infusions.[23]

Ketamine-assisted psychotherapy (KAP) has been used for over fifty years in the treatment of heroin, cocaine, and alcohol dependence, as well as food addiction. Thousands of patients have been detoxified from alcohol using ketamine with no reported complications.[24] Originally, KAP found unparalleled reductions in relapse rates in alcoholism; one year later, they found that 66 percent of these patients were still abstinent.[25] Morgan and others have shown that KAP achieves similar results.[26]

Many ask if KAP is better than AA for achieving alcohol abstinence. There are many pros and cons in considering such a question. First, AA is well-known and undoubtedly helps millions worldwide. However, the research on the effectiveness of AA is controversial and subject to widely divergent interpretations.[27] KAP is psychotherapy with a trained professional, usually a psychiatrist or psychologist. AA is done in large groups and delivered by laypeople. However, most people running the AA groups are ex-alcoholics themselves, so they know exquisitely well the road these people are traveling. There has never been a study utilizing KAP along with AA, but the idea is certainly intriguing.

Now that we have better-clarified addiction, we can delve into why a drug like ketamine helps addiction. Three stages define ketamine-assisted psychotherapy: the first stage is preparatory, during which patients undergo a preliminary psychotherapy session in which they are directed to view the world symbolically, realize the negative effects of alcohol dependence, and see the positive sides of sobriety. In the second stage, ketamine is administered, and the psychotherapist verbally guides the patient to create new meaning and purpose in life. At moments of a highly intense psychedelic experience, the smell of alcohol is introduced to the patients (this is because olfaction is directly connected with emotional areas in the brain). In the third stage, psychotherapy is performed after the session. With the help of a therapist, patients share their experiences with others the following day after the ketamine session.

Psychologist Jordan Peterson is quoted as saying, "The funny thing is you're trying to stop drinking alcohol, you've got to find something better than alcohol—and alcohol's pretty good! So you've got to find something better." The point is not to ask why people drink too much; rather, it is better to ask why they would stop. One reason ketamine and other psychedelics work is that they give people compassionate investigation into themselves. It helps us look at the trauma injury spectrum and allows us to uncover the blind spots.

All addiction arises from intolerable feelings never processed or dealt with. Dr. John Krystal says that ketamine affects alcohol-related memories by beneficially interfering with neuroplasticity and lessening the impact of those triggers and memories, leading to better decisions. We have three nervous systems in the human body—our brain, our heart, and our gastrointestinal system. What happens in the mind happens in the body. People discount these seemingly small "t" traumas until conjured up from the depths by therapy and psychedelics. We must see past the medical definition of addiction as a disease instead of a normal response to trauma. All the rhetoric of "just saying no" does not result in people making so-called better choices.

Ketamine helps you expose the truth of your life. This is key to understanding addiction and why a drug like ketamine can help. The drugs help people lose their inhibitions. Ketamine and other psychedelics open up mutually candid conversations, which is what helps. Imagine if ketamine or other psychedelics could be used in prisons, where more than half the population is addicted to a substance. Most felons who are released from prison return to the same addictive environments that helped land them in prison in the first place. According to the National Association of Drug Court Professionals, 95 percent of incarcerated addicts use drugs again after they are released and 60 to 80 percent will commit a new crime, often related to their drug addiction. What if ketamine or other psychedelics, along with psychotherapy, could help even a percentage of the population? Enormous amounts of strife and money could potentially be saved by decreasing crime and giving us more productive members of society.

Despite all this, most psychedelics, except ketamine, are not legal for use, despite many studies showing they are safe and effective for treating mental disorders. We struggle to get these substances legalized because of outdated and strenuous regulations created by government officials decades ago.

Ketamine and Eating Disorders

In 1998, Cambridge University researchers successfully treated severe patients with eating disorders and made national headline news.[28] They found that nine patients responded to ketamine treatments, showed prolonged remission from anorexia, and found it easier to maintain social contact and discuss future plans.

Psychedelics and eating disorders may seem an unlikely pair, but research is making a lot of headway in this very difficult-to-treat condition. Anorexia nervosa and bulimia are forms of compulsive behaviors in people with a perfectionist personality. The drive to reduce body weight has become beyond normal control in these patients. Psychotherapy as a sole treatment is frequently unsuccessful in the most severe cases. The most intense anorexics have constant relapses and seek several practitioners hoping for a magic cure. The severity of compulsive behaviors disrupts whole families.

Dr. Lori Calabrese published a study on using a ketogenic diet followed by ketamine treatments used specifically to treat anorexia nervosa.[29] The patient experienced complete and sustained remission of anorexia and weight restoration. Certainly, there are many unanswered questions about psychedelics and eating disorders, but the current research points to a positive trend in this challenging, sometimes catastrophic disease.

Caroline Beckwith provides a popular, honest account on YouTube recounting her riveting struggle with anorexia nervosa and how she used ketamine and a ketogenic diet to overcome her struggle.[30] She was anorexic before she even knew what anorexia was. She sought treatment at Johns Hopkins University without relief. She continued exercising seven days a week and frequently fasted, which she describes as a living hell. She adopted the ketogenic diet with some success. Then she read about the 1998 Cambridge study using ketamine and decided to try it herself. After four ketamine treatments, she found a way to get out of anorexia and left it behind for good.

CHAPTER SEVEN

Athletes, Mental Illness, and Suicide

"To show weakness, we're told, in so many words, is to deserve shame. But I am here to show weakness. And I am not ashamed."

—*Mardy Fish*

Michael Phelps once said, "For the longest time, I thought asking for help was a sign of weakness because that's kind of what society teaches us. Well, you know what? If someone wants to call me weak for asking for help, that's their problem. Because I'm saving my own life." Phelps's quote gives us a glimpse of how the athletics world perceives mental health.

Suicide is an important and preventable cause of death among athletes. Junior Seau, Wade Belak, and Jovan Belcher have the following in common: they all reached their dreams of becoming successful professional athletes and have ended their own lives for different reasons. Hundreds of athletes are opening up about mental illness in the NFL (football), UFC (mixed martial arts), NHL (hockey), MLB (baseball), ATP (tennis), and Olympic sports; all sports governing bodies have recently prioritized mental health concerns for athletes. Chronic traumatic encephalopathy (CTE), depression, and suicide make headline news nowadays. Many athletes are opening up and speaking about their experiences with psychotherapy and psychedelics and how they have helped them guide their careers and lives.

ESPN commentator and journalist Kate Fagan wrote a riveting book titled, *What Made Maddy Run*.[1] It is the story of a collegiate athlete, Madison Holleran, suffering from severe depression. She excelled in academics and was incredibly popular, genuinely kind and personable, and a collegiate track athlete at the University of Pennsylvania. On January 17, 2014, she ran off the rooftop of a parking garage near the university and fell to her death. Holleran's suicide rocked the University of Pennsylvania campus. In fact, in a span of ten years, the University of Pennsylvania has recorded at least fourteen student suicides, including Holleran.[2] College counseling centers became inundated with mental health crises, and the university responded by hiring additional counselors and cutting wait times. In 2019, Gregory Eells, the head of counseling and psychological services (CAPS) at Penn, died of suicide, highlighting the complexity of the school's continuing battle against suicide.[3]

The risk factors associated with depression in university undergraduate students are complex. Some of the risk factors include:[4]

- Low self-esteem and confidence
- Lack of social engagement
- Infrequent family visits
- Excessive internet and social media usage
- Belonging to minority groups
- Inadequate physical activity and obesity
- Loneliness
- Underlying mental health condition
- Studying in a foreign language
- Workload pressure
- Low family income/childhood poverty
- Eating disorders
- Tobacco, drug, and alcohol usage
- Being bullied by staff
- Gender
- Inadequate sleep
- Wrong expectations

- Subject mastery
- Exams and assessments
- Inadequate financial support from the university
- Lack of social support network
- Sexual victimization
- Year of study
- Unfamiliar environment
- Age

Athletes have all of those risk factors as well as living up to expectations from coaches, family, friends, and sponsors. Student-athletes face unique pressures that involve balancing training and games, homework, social life, tests, vacations, relationships, and social gatherings while developing into young adults. For example, a survey of nearly 3,000 students in five US universities showed that more than half experienced anxiety and depression.[5] Factors such as injury, failure, and drugs may lead to an increased risk of depression and suicidal behavior in anyone.[6]

Social media is gaining even more significance among high school and college athletes with the NCAA now allowing name, image, and likeness sponsorship deals. College athletes will undoubtedly be focusing on social media more than ever before. Fagan's book highlights Madison Holleran's social media activities and her attempts to appear perfect in a world she could not control. Even the images she posted sixty minutes before jumping were filtered with an ethereal quality.[7] Madison's life story reveals a unique perspective on the struggles of young college student-athletes suffering from mental illness. Madison seemingly effortlessly attained perfection in high school but could not obtain it at an Ivy League school where she was just one of many. The pressure was too much, and she became isolated, constantly fighting her battle with depression; her story reveals today's mounting pressures of being perfect in an age of relentless connectivity and social media overload. Madison was undergoing intense therapy before her suicide; if she had been able to undergo ketamine therapy for her severe depression, could the outcome have been different?

Everyone presents an edited version of life on social media, and shared moments reflect an ideal life. If you were to look up a definition of perfection, it would state, "lacking all faults or defects or satisfying all requirements." Young women growing up on Instagram spend inordinate amounts of time absorbing others' filtered images while paying less attention to the reality in front of them. Nobody posts the truth on social media; it's all smoke and mirrors. Instagram is passed off as real life but people filter their photos, brightening their images so as not to show the sadness they might genuinely feel.

Students and athletes alike may have many Instagram friends, but all they have mastered is the art of being alone in a crowded room without considering the cost. Psychologists Jonathan Haidt and Jean Twenge have been tracking the attitudes and behaviors of teens and young adults for years (Twenge), and they believe teens spend less time nowadays with their friends in person, and more using social media and other electronic means of communication. In many classrooms, students are entirely absorbed in their smartphones, sitting in complete silence. A *Journal of Adolescence* article showed that in 36 out of 37 countries, loneliness at school has increased since 2012.[8] Many students describe having shallow friendships and superfluous romantic relationships mediated by social media. In today's society, we can be two feet from a friend or loved one, yet those two people may as well be two thousand miles apart, and the irony is that both parties are lonely. People often have a thousand social media friends that they've never actually talked to, choosing instead to bounce one-line messages hundreds of times per day. Jonathan Haidt calls this "compare and despair"—you don't actually get social relationships, you get weak, fake social links. As Fagan says in her book, this is not friendship; this is a distraction.

The internet has addicted the world with a stimulus response, resulting in abnormal hyperactive reactions to the excitement and adrenaline rush. The biological effects of social media addiction are real. Research has clearly shown that children who instant messaged their mothers after undergoing a stressor did not release oxytocin and had salivary cortisol levels as high as those who did not interact with their parents. In contrast, children who interacted with their mothers in person or over the phone have increased oxytocin levels and decreased cortisol levels. Messaging appears comparable with not speaking with anyone at all.[9] Years of research has shown that oxytocin is the brain chemical essential in neuroendocrine mechanisms for social behavior and bonding and controls emotional connections.

Universities must continue efforts at destigmatizing mental health on campuses to enable students to receive more on-campus support. Students can shield themselves from isolation by participating in athletic and group activities such as club and collegiate sports, which can act as protective factors against depression. Students should use social media to stay in touch and interact with friends, family, and communities, not aim for perfection or a stage performance. Therefore, universities must allocate more resources to understanding the dangers of social media as well as support sporting and social activities that can impact students' mental health.[10]

Some athletes try to take their own lives, but the universe has other plans. The following story is about a professional baseball player, Drew Robinson, and his attempted suicide during the lockdowns and his path to choosing life.[11, 12]

* * * *

Case Study: Drew Robinson

On the morning of April 16, 2020, professional baseball player Drew Robinson sat at his kitchen table, finishing a note to his family explaining why he would end his life. This young man recently signed a major league baseball contract with the San Francisco Giants and should have felt on top of the world. Suicide knows no boundaries. Being confined by the lockdowns during the COVID-19 crisis for over a month undoubtedly led him closer to the decision. He hated his life; even worse, he hated that no one knew how much he hated his life. Hiding his hate and hopelessness, Drew was living his dream but still wanted to die.

Around 5:00 p.m., everything came together: a handgun, a neatly placed letter, a clean house, and some whiskey. He drove to the park in his truck. However, he decided he did not want to die in his truck, so he returned home. Three hours later, alone on his couch, he reached for his gun on the coffee table and discharged a bullet against his right temple.

Over the next twenty hours, he realized his suicide was the beginning of another story. Shortly after the gunshot, Drew looked around, confused that he was still conscious. Disappointed as one could be who wanted to commit suicide, he lay down on the ground and waited to die. Thirty minutes passed. He held a rag to his head, as one would instinctively do to cover their wounds. It did not hurt. He took a shower, then fell and lay on the bathroom floor. Later, he found himself lying in his bed. He even tried to brush his teeth. He remembered thinking to himself how ridiculous it all was. He had a hole in his head and was brushing his teeth. Four hours after pulling the trigger, he was alive, but still planned to let himself bleed.

The following day, he woke up in pain to the sound of his phone buzzing. He went to the kitchen, drank water, and took a Tylenol. The gun was still on the coffee table, but he grabbed his phone instead. He stared at his reflection in the bathroom mirror and did not recognize his face. He again saw his gun on the coffee table and thought about baseball. He wondered, "Could I play with one eye?" He wondered if thinking about the future meant he was trying to survive.

That single Tylenol pill. Was it some subconscious message that he wanted to live? Drew looked at his phone and saw a text from his friend Darryl, who had come over to work out in his gym. In the afternoon, Drew returned to the couch where it all started, with the gun and his cell phone on the coffee table. Holding the gun to his head a second time, he dialed 911 and asked for an ambulance.

It was 3:44 p.m. when Drew called 911, wondering how on earth he was still alive.

"I need an ambulance," he said. "I tried to commit suicide last night, and I made it through. I think I detached my eye, maybe. I can't open it, and I have a huge hole in my head, and I'm in a lot of pain."

"What'd you do?" the dispatcher asked.

"I shot myself in the head," Drew said.

Police in the area rushed to his house.

At 3:51 p.m., police kicked down the front door. They were afraid this might be an ambush. A guy shoots himself in the head and lives for twenty hours?

At 3:52 p.m., the officer asked: "Why'd you shoot yourself?" Drew replied in a whisper: "Because I hate myself."

At 3:53 p.m., an ambulance arrived and transported Drew to the UMC Trauma Center.

At 4:00 p.m., the police officer shook his head and said what everyone else was thinking: "That's crazy that he's still alive."

How did Drew live for nearly twenty-four hours with a gunshot wound to his head? And without medical attention? Few survive self-inflicted gunshot wounds to the head like this. American construction worker Phineas Gage survived an iron rod driven through his head. However, Gage's friends remarked that he was "no longer Gage." Drew was lucky. He emerged from his experience better, with renewed purpose, clarity, and confidence.

Drew's right eye was beyond repair. The human eye is a remarkably resilient structure that is surrounded by bones, muscles, and fat. The orbital cavity provides ample protection from everyday life but not from a 9 mm bullet traveling at Mach speed. The fracture in his frontal sinus caused the fluid from his brain to leak, posing a significant infection risk. The bullet missed the major arteries, his left orbital floor, and exited above his left cheekbone.

The doctors had to reconstruct Drew's face. The first procedure was surgery to save his right eyelid. The second was to reconstruct the eye orbit and to return most of the symmetry to his face. The third was to fix the fracture in his sinuses and stop the cerebrospinal fluid leakage, which, if left untreated, could have led to meningitis, brain abscesses, chronic headaches, and death. The final and fourth surgery was an enucleation, the removal of Drew's right eye. He lost his senses of taste and smell after the surgeries.

Life is unrelenting. Today, Drew knows mental-health issues are challenging to discuss; regardless, he wants to share his experience with others that mental illness is winnable. He feels he was supposed to go through a suicide attempt.

"I shot myself," he says. "But I killed my ego. I'm free now."

Drew does not glorify what happened. He knows he should be dead. Instead, he is focused on fixing himself and his surrounding relationships while maintaining a professional baseball career. He prefers not to wear his eye prosthesis to show the world what he did and have more opportunities to share his experiences. Drew believes that "I was supposed to tell a story." When Drew eventually spoke with his brother Chad, he repeated, "I'm meant to be alive, Chad. I'm meant to be alive. I'm meant to be alive. I'm here for a reason. I want to tell the world what happened so I can heal, and maybe I can help others heal, too."

Drew explains, "How can I go through this and not find a way to try to help other people? To have this happen and move on with my life the way I was before? There's no way. This was an enormous sign that I'm supposed to help people get through something they don't think is winnable."

The contributing factors to Drew's decision to attempt suicide are apparent if you study his family history. When Drew's parents, Renee and Darryl, were divorcing, it devastated him. After the divorce, the Robinson family splintered. The boys went to live with Darryl while his sister Britney stayed with Renee. They found common ground in one place: the baseball field. He remembers asking himself questions. "Is there something wrong with me? Why is Mom so mad at me? What did I do?" The Robinsons didn't discuss those sorts of things. They just lived one day to the next. The family never handled emotions well, causing stress and internal struggles. "I think we all had this idea of a perfect family and things like that. When it didn't live up to that, we questioned everything we were doing."

Drew's brother, Chad, was drafted to the Milwaukee Brewers in 2006, setting a near-impossible standard in Drew's mind. Drew became obsessed with an image of perfection. He made varsity at Silverado High School as a freshman and became the best player there since his brother. Professional sports put tremendous pressure on Drew. There were the 4:30 a.m. wake-up calls for workouts, long bus rides, injuries, and drug testing. Being a professional baseball player isn't only about playing baseball better than everyone else. It is an accelerated adulthood for eighteen-year-old, paying bills, managing disappointment, navigating politics, forging relationships, and figuring out how to live in a universe designed to weed out the weak.

Drew's life seemed ideal: he had a professional baseball contract, family support, and a fiancée. Despite all these positives, Drew could not stop hating himself. Despite powerful support from his fiancée, Daiana, he broke off the relationship abruptly. She thought they were going to get married, and just like that, it was over. Drew was stuck in a rut with never-ending questions in his mind:

"Why does everything suck? Why is this happening to me? Is there something I'm doing wrong? Why can't you just be honest with everyone and let them know how much you hate yourself? Is it even worth it? Is my life even worth it?"

His self-doubt paralyzed his life. He never felt like he belonged. The voice in his head grew louder and more depressed. His suicidal ideation intensified. Understanding that he needed help, he saw a therapist and read self-development books. He wanted to see himself the way he perceived everyone else saw themselves. But the self-doubt compounded into another question:

"Who would care if I'm gone?"

When no answer came, he planned his suicide. Drew visited a gun range in the Phoenix area, and each shot birthed another question.

"Could this be a real possibility? How would I even do it? Where would I do it? No," Drew then told himself. "No! That's too extreme. Just talk to someone and get some help. We can do it. Just talk to someone. Find anyone, even if it's a surface-level conversation. Nobody wants to hear it. Nobody needs to hear it."

He continued therapy sessions, but they didn't rid him of his worst thoughts. His frustration with himself multiplied. He was trying to embrace his vulnerability, but even if Daiana and others saw progress, he saw stasis. He began to feel he wasn't good enough for her and hated himself. He called off the wedding.

Then COVID-19 shut down the baseball world in March. Drew returned to Las Vegas to an empty house, lonely and no longer knowing who he was. A week later, he purchased a gun and returned on March 30 to pick it up. He had no surface-level conversations or light-hearted camaraderie to sway his resolve. Drew could no longer meet with friends or go to the stadium, and he was alone with the negative thoughts built up over two decades.

The days seemed to last forever. Friends checked in with Drew, wanting to plan something for his twenty-eighth birthday on April 20. He ignored them. On April 13, Drew met with a woman who had a litter of puppies. He petted and cuddled one. Then a heavy feeling weighed down on him. "Sorry," he told the woman. "I can't take this dog." He left hurriedly, noticing the confused look on the woman's face. "She had no idea," Drew remembers. "How could she? I couldn't take the dog because I was planning on killing myself."

Survivors of suicide attempts, particularly ones as violent as Drew's, have a wide range of outcomes. The combination of physical and mental trauma typically requires a reset of the body and mind that takes years. When he emerged from anesthesia after the initial surgery, Drew said he felt love for the blanket warming him, for each breath that filled his lungs, and for his family. Never had he felt compelled to say he loved them. Saying "I love you" was just a habit, what you're supposed to say. Drew was determined that his "after" would be different from his "before."

"I never will hold back from asking or telling someone, even if it's something simple," Drew says. "Hey, this little thing's annoying me today. Just tell them. They want to hear it. People who love you want to hear it; if you don't have people who love you, therapists want to hear it. People want to help you. So many people in this world will help anyone go through these things. It might be a specific situation that makes you feel you're alone, but you're never alone. Think about it. Not everyone can do it. So, if not everyone can do it, but some people can, that's just like having strength. Hey, I reached out to someone today. I told him how I felt, and I felt really good. Why can't that be a strength?"

Drew had found that strength emerging from those twenty dark hours, from the shadowy details he somehow remembered when he reconsidered his family and the idea of coming back to play baseball, not just to see if he could, but to show others what is possible.

Cleaning Drew's house after the suicide attempt was something parents should never have to experience. They were entering through the garage and unprepared for what they saw. His mother looked up the phone numbers of hazmat cleaners.

"No," Darryl responded. "We're cleaning it." No way was he going to let a stranger into the house to see the remnants of his son's worst moment. Darryl scoured the walls while Chad wiped the floors, and Britney handled the linens. She borrowed an industrial carpet cleaner from her office. They were on their hands and knees, knowing they couldn't erase reality, but determined to scrub as much of it away as possible.

Drew needed to experience the house where he almost died. He walked toward the couch and sat in the same spot where he shot himself.

"I wanted to feel it again," he says. "I wanted to feel the power, not the bad side. I'm still here." When Daiana, Darryl, Britney, and Chad visited him at the house that night, he walked them through the twenty hours. They were speechless. "No one understands how I made it through," he says. "No one has to." He said they could ask him anything.

"They each wanted to know, 'what could we have done?'"

'Nothing. It was my responsibility, not yours.'

'How come we didn't know?'

'Because I was good at hiding my sadness.'

'Why did you do it?'"

Drew didn't have a good response to this one. He remembered what he told the police officer: that he hated himself.

Suicide attempts leave behind the sort of choppy wake that can waylay even a person who has had years of therapy and proper medication. People who attempt suicide often try it again until they succeed. "I don't have it all figured out, but I'm working on it," Drew says. "It's not something that you just achieve. You don't just achieve self-growth. You don't get to a point where you just have it and don't have to work at it again. You don't get to a point; oh, I'm happy today. That's it. I'm going to be happy for the rest of my life. It's the same way in the opposite. I had a rough day. That doesn't mean the rest of your life will suck."

Drew follows a daily regimen. He typically wakes before his alarm. He plays with his dogs, Ellie and Brodi, and then goes into the kitchen, drinks a jug of water, and meditates for twenty minutes. He then goes to the gym, eats breakfast, and goes to the office—one day at a time.

In the afternoon, Drew tries to make at least three phone calls to connect, catch up, ask questions, and talk about how he's doing. He'll work out again, either in his gym or at the batting cages, before returning home to listen to music, watch TV, or spend time with his family. Before bed, Drew does some journaling. Sometimes he'll write a whole page, and sometimes just a sentence. Either way, every entry ends with the same eight words:

"I LOVE MYSELF, AND I LOVE MY LIFE!!"

Drew's mission in life has changed substantially. After leaving the hospital, Drew remained in contact with the Giants' management. He sent them pictures and videos of himself in the gym and field. The Giants psychologist put pieces of tape with the names of each nurse at UMC hospital on Drew's jersey on National Front-Line Workers' Day. September 10 is World Suicide Prevention Day, and Drew asked if he could speak to his teammates, the Giants' players, and staff. Playing baseball was important, but if Drew was going to help others, he needed to tell his story. The Giants welcomed the idea. He arrived at Oracle Park wearing a mask with a Giants logo and no eye prosthesis. The players, coaches, and other staff gathered outside. Drew spoke with the microphone and said, "First, I just want to say thank you for everything. What I've been going through the last couple of months has been the most powerful experience. The lessons I've learned from what I've gone through are something I want to share.

"On April 16th, around 8:00 p.m., I attempted suicide and shot myself in the head. A day later, on April 17th, around 4:00 p.m., I dialed 911 myself in an attempt to have my life saved. Later that night, my life was not only saved but reborn and restarted."

Drew spoke about the importance of talking, the need for others, and his intention to give baseball another shot. He saw people crying, and some were undoubtedly thinking of family or friends lost to suicide.

In November, a familiar feeling seized Drew. Something was off. It started with a skipped workout, then a missed meditation session and journal entry. The pressures of his new routine and the new expectations he had set were getting to him. His mind racing, Drew told himself he was lazy and wasn't doing the work to stay healthy. "If I can't do the work, why would I deserve happiness? If I can't even do enough to earn happiness, what's the point?" He didn't leave his room for a day. One day turned into two, and then three. His negative self-talk sounded like the Drew "before," not the Drew "after." "I just felt like the world was ending," he says. "I had my first passive suicidal thought, which scared me: I wish I'd been successful." Sticking to his daily routine, continuing to see his therapist, Dr. Zand, and believing in his mission helped him through this challenging period.

Drew will never know what caused him to call 911 that day, but the clues have always been there. In the hours before he pulled the trigger, and throughout those twenty hours, his thoughts constantly converged on his family and then fiancée Daiana. Reminders of April 16 now surround him. Drew kept the shorts he was wearing, the blood-soaked towel, and the note he had written to his family. His parents removed the plank of wood where the bullet had lodged and made it into a necklace for him.

Today, Drew Robinson has traded his baseball glove for a microphone and is an anti-suicide advocate for the BetterUcare.com foundation, where he is the spokesperson and cofounder. He raises awareness for suicide prevention with a social media platform, along with psychiatrist Dr. Sam Zand and Hollywood actor and entrepreneur Derek Du Chesne.

Source: Personal interview with Drew Robinson and adapted from ESPN article, "San Francisco Giants outfielder Drew Robinson's remarkable second act." May 11, 2020. Jeff Passan on ESPN E:60 Preview.

* * * *

Mental Health, Suicide, and Psychedelics Among Athletes

Athletes are imperfect role models for both physical and mental health. The term "unhealthy athlete" sounds a bit like a paradox. An athlete can be fit but unhealthy both physically and mentally. Clearly, athletes have lower rates of heart disease, stroke, and smoking-related cancers. Images of athletes performing portray the perception of perfect health, but internal fitness is more important than the veneer. Our culture celebrates harder, faster, stronger, and the ethos of "just play through it." Mental health is seldom spoken about in professional sports. Athletes often experience disordered eating, depression, insomnia, mood disorders, loss of motivation, reduced mental concentration, and anxiety. On the physical side, athletes often overtrain themselves. The stakes are often high, and professional and amateur athletes are not known for prioritizing their mental health. The mantra that struggling teammates are weak is common in college and professional sports. Even more, signs of mental weakness strike fear into athletes because they might not be able to do their job and risk being replaced in a highly competitive environment. Subsequently, athletes fear the stigma of "being soft." Solomon Thomas of the Las Vegas Raiders says, "It's like you are being judged for everything you do; guys are cut, traded, and signed every day. As much as you want to say it should be different, it's hard because you might open up to someone one day, and they're gone."

Although hundreds of athletes suffer from mental illness, not enough have opened up about it; some notable examples of NFL athletes who have are Darren Waller, Solomon Thomas, D. J. Chark, Demario Davis, Aaron Rodgers, A. J. Brown, Calvin Ridley, and Adam Thielen.[13] In professional tennis, Naomi Osaka appeared on the cover of *Time* with the text reading, "IT'S O.K. TO NOT BE O.K." She opened up about her struggles with depression and anxiety before the 2021 French Open, from which she withdrew.[14] The former US Open champion Bianca Andreescu announced she would not compete at the Australian Open, citing depression and sadness due to the frequent lockdowns during COVID. In July 2021, Olympic gymnast Simone Biles withdrew from the finals, citing "the twisties," a heightened state of anxiety.[15]

Many athletes, such as Michael Phelps and Terry Bradshaw, have come out after their careers about their bouts of depression and suicidality. Numerous athletes fall into depression after their careers are ended. Boxing legend Sugar Ray Leonard famously said, "Nothing could satisfy me out of the ring." Leonard's struggles with retirement and severe depression were well documented. Some professional athletes even commit suicide after their careers. One such example was professional cyclist Jonathan Cantwell.

Athletes and Addiction

Athletics and mental health are closely connected. Addiction is a complex mind, body, and brain disorder that doesn't have a single cause. Athletes are often primed for addiction, and research has shown that sports increase the risk factors for addiction. A common trait among athletes is hyper-competitiveness, a risk factor for addictive behaviors. Athletes strive to be the best at whatever they do, including being the best heroin user if that's their drug of choice.

The environment athletes are placed in promulgates addiction. Athletes are constantly adored by fans and the media. They are pampered and repeatedly told that they are the best and their actions, right or wrong, are positively affirmed. Athletes form strong social bonds, affiliations, and a tribal mentality, especially in team sports. Many professional athletes harbor a false notion of "being chosen" to do their respective sport and are devoted to being famous or known. Everyone is paying attention to the athlete.

From a biological perspective, the neurotransmitter dopamine is one reason for athletes' success, but it also partially explains why they may become addicted to drugs, sex, and gambling. We know that dopamine plays a role in addiction, but it's one piece of a massive puzzle. Athletes are constantly looking for dopamine. It's the same rush a child receives repeatedly playing video games or the feeling an emotional eater obtains after devouring an entire box of pastries, but an athlete's life is one of searching for the rush they get with each subsequent success. Whether in practice or competition, the athletes' journey is filled with peaks and valleys of dopamine. When the career ends, the dopamine hits end with it, leaving the brain asking for more.

Dopamine is one reason substance abuse is entrenched in sports culture; glaring examples are the locker rooms and bars filled with alcohol after a victory. Painkillers and other drugs are readily available, including performance-enhancing drugs. Drugs and alcohol are surprisingly available to adolescent athletes. This is especially relevant with the advent of high school and collegiate players now being paid exorbitant amounts of money to play sports. A recent example is high school football star Nico Iamaleava who reportedly signed a deal worth 8 million dollars to play for the University of Tennessee at Knoxville.

While dopamine isn't the sole cause of addiction, its motivational properties certainly play a role. For all of their careers, they receive dopamine rush after dopamine rush. For instance, sex addiction has little to do with a high sex drive and everything to do with dopamine. Being a pro athlete is a dopamine addiction, and this dopamine roller coaster predisposes athletes to mental illness and even suicide.

One athlete who overcame major addiction is Darren Waller of the Las Vegas Raiders. Before becoming one of the NFL's best tight ends, Waller battled through drug addiction that started in high school. During an interview, he told me that he drank alcohol daily and took MDMA, Xanax, cocaine, and Oxycontin painkillers. Surprising even himself, he made it to the NFL, where he was spending hundreds a day on drugs; he failed multiple drug tests and was banned for a year. In 2017, he had a near-death experience after taking fentanyl. He entered rehab, and since August 11, 2017, he has never touched another drug. Waller is involved with several foundations that deal with addiction and are trying to make a change. He is also part of the Better U Foundation, a health startup trying to help eradicate the stigma of mental illness.[16]

Ketamine and the Elite Athletes

It's difficult to say if psychedelics can enhance sports performance. No one has studied it to any extent, and psychedelics are still returning from their sixty-year hiatus. Interestingly, the use of psychedelics in sports dates back to at least the 1970s when Doc Ellis, a pitcher for the Pittsburgh Pirates, threw a no-hitter against the San Diego Padres while on LSD and other substances. Endurance athletes, surfers, rock climbers, and extreme sports athletes have used psychedelics for years.[17, 18] Many exclaim that psychedelics "put them in the zone or a mythical heightened state." Psychedelics provoke an immersed engagement with any activity, allowing the athlete to analyze the movements and patterns in ways impossible while not under the influence. The enhancement is more psychological than physiological.

Former UFC champion Miesha Tate questions how psychedelics might affect some athletes.[19] She highlights that many athletes view sports as a coping mechanism or a "healthy" addiction. In this sense, athletes feed off of their mental issues, which helps them to compartmentalize their situations and gives them the incredible focus and determination it takes to win a championship; it also helps them to be nervous at the right moments to be successful. When Miesha beat Holly Holmes for the world championship, she was competing at her best. She remembers that fighting was an obsession and simultaneously her coping mechanism, which helped her overcome adversity and ultimately led her to become a champion. Admittedly, she recognizes that this type of mental outlook is ideal for being a successful athlete but probably not optimal for long-term mental health. Her hesitation in using psychedelics while competing is that it could take away that relentless edge many athletes depend on to drive forward toward their goals. She points out that psychedelics make you feel much more at peace with yourself and questions what effect this may have on the athlete. Perhaps peace has a price. Could it be that if psychedelics help an athlete with mental issues, they would also take away the intense drive to succeed? These are difficult questions, and no studies are out there to answer them. Indeed, every situation is unique, and every athlete falls on different parts of the mental health spectrum. For example, many athletes perform better when they start a family and have children. Likewise, some athletes perform better when they have overcome their addictions to drugs and alcohol; some do not. On paper, it seems like Naomi Osaka performed better when dealing with her depression versus when she started getting help and took time off the sport. In the case of motocross champion Zach Osborne, a sure sign that he was going to do well was when he was nervous and throwing up just before the gate dropped at the starting line.

Dr. Michael Miletic is a renowned psychiatrist and former Olympic weightlifter. He specializes in ketamine IV-assisted psychotherapy for athletes. As a former professional athlete, he understands the nuance that perseverance is often born out of trauma. He says that most athletes are unaware of their traumas or the need to adapt to them. In his experience, ketamine has the power to safely open up traumas that would be otherwise too painful to face and helps to begin a new life, free from all the constraints of the built-up unconscious traumas. With so much trauma fueling athletic performance and bringing untold suffering and emotional struggle, he looks forward to the day when professional sports not only allow but support ketamine and other psychedelic treatments for athletes.

He tells the story of a twenty-four-year-old NFL player who significantly benefited from ketamine IV-assisted psychotherapy. The ketamine sessions were initially challenging, but he ultimately returned to how he once felt as a young boy before his mother's death and how he once felt on the football field before becoming injured. Dr. Miletic says that the athlete is doing well today and still playing in the NFL. The complete story can be found on Dr. Miletic's blog at https://themileticcenter.com/ketamine-and-the-elite-athlete.

Depression and Suicide in Athletes

Jonathan Cantwell, an Australian professional cyclist, was born in 1982 in Brisbane, Australia. Cantwell reached the highest level of professional cycling during a career spanning over ten years. A loving and outgoing individual, he lived to race his bike, socialize, and meet people. Near the end of his career, Cantwell experienced many difficulties—his brother committed suicide, he divorced his wife, and he was fighting a legal battle with his cycling team. His brother's suicide was deeply traumatic. After his brother's death, he announced on social media that he would take care of his brother's kids. Jonathan's father also killed himself when Jonathan was young. Shortly after his career finished, Jonathan successfully battled testicular cancer and was cured. Like many ex-professional athletes, finding his new purpose in life proved difficult. He became CEO of a bike brand, hoping to make a name selling bikes, and he also started competing in triathlons.

In November 2018, Jonathan killed himself with a noose in his native Australia. Was his suicide due to genetics or specific life events? He certainly had a strong family history of suicide. Indeed, studies show that first-degree relatives of individuals who have committed suicide have more than twice the probability of killing themselves than the general population.[20]

Some scientists believe that suicidality is approximately 40 percent heritable, and the role of the environment makes up the rest. A closer examination of Jonathan's environmental factors would suggest that he was coming off a successful career and faced many legal and marital difficulties. For Jonathan, like so many ex-professional athletes, it was hard not knowing what to do next to get that next dopamine hit. It's not likely he took his life because he had a genetic predisposition. Instead, everything culminated around him to satisfy his conditions for suicide at a dark, vulnerable moment. Once again, we have to consider that if Jonathan could have received the proper treatment with ketamine and psychotherapy, he would still be here, laughing and joking nonstop like he always did. Unfortunately, the world will never know.

Today, more athletes are taking a stance on mental health, highlighting the need to optimize their views on life. Athletes often have multiple coaches: strength, conditioning, nutrition, physical therapy, and sports psychology. Athletes are speaking openly about using therapy, psychedelics, and medications to treat mental health conditions such as depression, anxiety, PTSD, addiction, and traumatic brain injury.[21]

Chronic traumatic encephalopathy, or CTE, is a brain condition associated with repeated impacts on the head. A definitive diagnosis can only be made in an autopsy, but a 2017 study showed that 99 percent of former NFL players and 91 percent of college football players have CTE. Depression and suicidality are central symptoms of CTE; others include memory loss, confusion, personality changes, and erratic behavior. Athletes who have had CTE and committed suicide include Junior Seau, Mike Webster, Aaron Hernandez, and Shane Dronett.

Former athletes including heavyweight champion Mike Tyson (boxing), Daniel Carcillo (NHL), Kerry Rhodes (NFL), Lamar Odom (NBA), and UFC fighters Ian McCall and Dean Lister are part of a growing movement of people using ketamine, plant medicines like ayahuasca, and psychedelic mushrooms to help heal PTSD and the symptoms of brain trauma. In November 2020, Bryant Gumbel began HBO's *Real Sports* segment with former NHL player Daniel Carcillo describing his suicide plan after retiring from hockey and his journey into psychedelics.[22] Diagnosed with seven concussions throughout his twelve-year professional hockey career, Carcillo says he likely experienced "hundreds more" and explored numerous avenues to address his mental health issues. After trying psychotherapy and antidepressants, he opted for something outside Western medicine's realm of treatment: ayahuasca, a South American brew revered by indigenous cultures as a powerful medicine containing the psychedelic compound N, N-Dimethyltryptamine, or DMT. "I'm just trying to look for more peace of mind, less suffering," he says to the cameras from the Peruvian jungle before attending the ceremony. Four hours later, he emerges feeling changed and calls it "the most amazing experience" of his life. Months later, when HBO's production team visits Carcillo, he says he's experiencing "little to no depression and anxiety." His symptoms included slurred speech, headaches, head pressure, memory issues, concentration, and insomnia—they are all completely gone. His wife exclaimed, "I didn't see him smile for years." With her husband still symptom-free after five months, she asks, "How can you not believe this stuff works?"

Another segment of *Real Sports* takes viewers inside a private ceremony where a group of fighters, including grappler and former UFC stars Dean Lister and Ian McCall, are guided through a psilocybin experience by a shaman. Ian McCall fought in the UFC and other professional MMA leagues for fifteen years before finally tapping out. Multiple injuries left him taking daily opiate painkillers, including fentanyl, turning him into a self-described "monster." Experimenting with psychedelics helped cure him of his addiction and suicidal thoughts. Today, he is committed to helping improve the mental health of other former fighters by showing them how beneficial life-altering group experiences with psychedelic medicines can be. "Fighters are good people," McCall says, "but they're tormented."

Dean Lister has experienced his fair share of head traumas, like any longtime mixed martial artist. He describes the symptoms associated with repeated concussions as being "stuck in a prison cell in your mind." Before taking five grams of psilocybin mushrooms, Lister struggled with alcoholism, drinking up to twenty beers daily and taking Xanax every night. During the deep journey (the only kind afforded to anyone who consumes five grams, aka a hero's dose), Lister hallucinated that he was having a near-death experience and said to himself, "If I wake up, I'm going to do things differently." Since the experience, he's steered clear of all drugs and alcohol.

Undoubtedly, psychedelics like ketamine can save lives for those ex-professional athletes who are severely depressed and have suicidal ideations. Indeed, as more research is published on psychedelics over the coming years, a clearer picture of these drugs' overall effects will emerge. Mike Tyson claims psychedelics saved his life. He was suicidal and depressed as his life was riddled with emotional instability, drug addiction, and legal troubles. After his psychedelic experiences, he exclaims, "I will never be the same again. Fight your fears, and don't be afraid to try them. You can't be free unless you free yourself from fear."

Since then, the number of athletes emerging from the psychedelic closet has grown. NFL quarterback Aaron Rodgers spoke openly about his ayahuasca experience on *The Joe Rogan Experience*. Motocross racer Adam Cianciarulo described his ayahuasca retreat on the *Pulp MX Show*. They both describe the experience as challenging but did it for spiritual and emotional reasons and to help with life and professional aspirations. Both depicted it as a remarkable experience and a restorative reset. Athletes who have healed using ketamine therapy include NBA player Lamar Odom and NFL player Kenny Stills.[23] In addition to psychotherapy, many of these players report increased empathy and love for others, self-joy, and life from a different perspective. Stills says, "What ketamine does is it kind of takes away these extra levels of anxiety and the different processes happening in the brain so that we can be our true selves." An Australian research paper says that there is evidence that psychedelic-assisted psychotherapy appears to be capable of safe, long-lasting, and meaningful changes under certain conditions. As sports reach higher levels of precision, athletes will undoubtedly look for any advantage, including taking psychedelics for sports performing enhancement. Currently, the World Anti-Doping Agency (WADA) does not explicitly prohibit the use of psychedelics in sports, as they do not assume these substances are performance-enhancing. Time will tell.

CHAPTER EIGHT

How Ketamine Overcomes Mental Illness and Suicide

"A sad soul can kill you quicker than a germ."

—*John Steinbeck*

Ketamine is the most vital breakthrough in mental illness in decades. With suicides at their highest number in thirty years and 21 million adults experiencing an episode of major depression in 2020,[1] medical experts agree that rapid treatment for depression and suicide is highly desirable.[2] Considering the limitations in the clinical management of acute suicidal ideation, using ketamine has gained interest worldwide.

Standard treatments for suicide and depression include antidepressants, electro-convulsive therapy (ECT), psychotherapy, cognitive behavior therapy, lithium, and clozapine.[3, 4] Each of these longstanding treatment modalities has established efficacy for reducing markers of depression and suicidality, but no chemical or physical treatment for depression has been totally successful.[5] Unfortunately, over 50 percent of patients will be resistant to any one treatment approach.[6] Medications take weeks to work, and psychotherapy continues to be the mainstay of treatment. Truthfully, the treatment of mental illness has not changed much in fifty years and none of these therapies have moved the bar very far in preventing suicides.

Pharmaceutical companies have not invested in research for new psychiatric medicines since the 1950s, when researchers accidentally discovered that tuberculosis medications, isoniazid and iproniazid, suddenly caused depressed patients to become more cheerful, optimistic, and physically active, thus improving depression and curing tuberculosis.[7, 8]

The mechanism of how ketamine works in the brain differs from traditional antidepressants, and it certainly works faster. The studies advocating ketamine in stopping suicide have been largely ignored by the media, although that is changing. Hopefully, by 2025, ketamine will become the standard of care in emergency departments in the treatment of suicidal ideation, helping most to avoid institutionalization and saving millions in healthcare dollars.[9]

"Ketamine is the most important breakthrough in antidepressant treatment in decades," said Thomas Insel, MD, the former head of the National Institute of Mental Health. Ketamine is a dissociative anesthetic. It is currently a class III scheduled drug (approved for hospital or medical settings). At high doses, ketamine is an ideal anesthetic. In low doses, it causes an altered perception of sight and sound, pain relief, and dissociative and hallucinatory effects in humans. Perhaps better known in the rave scene and veterinary anesthesia, ketamine is one of the most enigmatic findings in modern psychiatry research.

Antidepressants require four to eight weeks to affect depression and suicidal ideation, and ketamine could fill that time gap or even serve as a single agent. Ketamine can be beneficial, even life-saving, for anyone going through suicidal ideations or suffering from severe depression. Many studies have shown the beneficial, rapid effects of ketamine, even after a single treatment. The lifting of depression persists even when the ketamine has exited your system.

Ketamine differs from other psychiatric medications. It is a rapidly acting drug that can prevent suicidal behaviors and the associated extreme emotional pain. A single sub-anesthetic dose of ketamine can reduce depression and stop suicidal ideation.[10] Aside from case reports about ketamine, there have been many randomized, double-blind, placebo-controlled studies involving large numbers of patients. Notably, many of these studies have been successfully repeated. However, like antidepressants, not all patients respond.[11] In those patients who respond, a ketamine infusion quickly results in antidepressant effects and abates impulsive suicidal thoughts.

Recent studies are showing the anti-suicidal effects of ketamine are independent of the antidepressant response. Since ketamine's discovery, significant efforts have been made to disentangle its complex molecular mechanisms and find broader clinical applicability. Ketamine and other psychedelics change what happens in the brain. In one study, subjects underwent a ketamine infusion, and their brain activity was imaged using a special MRI called a functional MRI (fMRI). People with depression revealed more normal fMRI activity in the PFC following ketamine administration.[12] Ketamine seems to help people become "unstuck" from abnormal patterns of brain activity associated with repetitive, negative thoughts. The same study was replicated in patients with suicidal thoughts. Four hours after the ketamine infusion, the PFC hyperactivity calmed down, which correlates with fewer thoughts of suicide. In this sense, ketamine may be akin to using a "defibrillator on the brain," putting it back into normal rhythm. The antidepressant mechanism of ketamine is unclear but likely involves glutamate and blocking NMDA receptors. Other SSRI medications, such as Fluoxetine and Citalopram, have also been shown to block NMDA receptors. Through the inhibition of NMDA receptors, ketamine allows the formation of new brain cell connections, a process called neuroplasticity.[13]

Suicide Treatment in the 21st Century

Suicide is unique in that either treatment is successful, or the result is the individual's death. Due to its impulsive and violent nature, suicide is difficult to study. For one, validating a person's response during a suicide attempt is difficult, if not impossible. Also, treating a suicidal person with a placebo medication would be unethical.

A variety of methods have been used to evaluate suicidal ideation. Most studies are accomplished in academic settings, but recent studies are from private practice. Psychiatrist Dr. Lori Calabrese performed one of the most extensive real-world studies involving 235 cases, where ketamine infusions eliminated suicidal ideation.[14] She showed that over 80 percent of patients with suicidal ideation could decrease or eliminate their suicidal ideation after serial ketamine infusions. Four weeks after the treatments, she found that none of the patients had attempted suicide, visited the emergency room, or had been hospitalized. Most patients needed three or more infusions to put their depression and suicidal ideation into remission. All the people in her clinic were treated with ketamine and received therapy involving a board-certified psychiatrist.

The National Institute of Health (NIH) studied the effect of a single treatment using ketamine on two groups: "wish to live" and "wish to die."[15] They found a significant number of the "wish to die" group switched to "wish to live." Ketamine specifically affects the desire to attempt suicide, independent of depression, suggesting that suicidal behavior might be distinct from depression.

A 2009 study was the first of its kind to publish ketamine's effects on suicidality in twenty-six patients in a psychiatric hospital setting.[16] Twenty-four hours after a single ketamine infusion, they observed substantial reductions in suicidal ideation. These researchers also saw a 50 percent decrease in overall Montgomery-Asberg Depression Rating Scale (MADRS) scores in those patients who received additional ketamine infusions.

The OKTOS (Oral Ketamine Trial on Suicidality) trial showed that oral ketamine reduces suicidal ideation.[17, 18] Though further study is needed, the idea that we can treat a person with suicidal ideation with oral ketamine opens the possibility of treating millions of people who have limited access to care or live in rural communities. This study also supports the recent increase in psychedelic telemedicine clinics that support a niche population.

In 2017, researcher Lucinda Grande described using oral ketamine to reduce suicidal behavior in two patients with a major depressive disorder.[19] Ketamine was added to their treatment regime, and they were monitored closely by phone and clinic visits over the next month. Both were given sublingual ketamine with instructions to take repeated doses every 1–2 hours until settled. The first patient, a man in his sixties, described an increasing "sense of calm" after his second dose. Half an hour later, he was markedly improved, smiling and joking. He returned to work a week later and discontinued ketamine after a month. The second patient was a man diagnosed with bipolar disorder and depression. He had a history of attempted suicide. Grande prescribed him a daily dose of ketamine over six months. The patient reported a reduction in suicidal thoughts. Though small, these case reports strongly suggest repeated and relatively low doses of oral ketamine can rapidly reduce suicidal thinking.

In palliative care, ketamine presents a valuable and safe option.[20] Patients with cancer have double the usual rate of suicide in the first two months of diagnosis. In 2016, Wei Fan published a study in which forty-two patients with newly diagnosed cancer, depression, and suicidal thoughts were given a single intravenous dose of ketamine and saw significant improvement following the infusion.[21]

Esketamine: The First New Antidepressant in Twenty Years

Janssen Pharmaceuticals recently brought to market the S-form of ketamine called Esketamine, naming it Spravato. Traditional ketamine is a racemic mixture consisting of equal parts of the S and R forms. They developed Esketamine because it has a higher potency than racemic ketamine, is more patient-friendly, and increases the possibility for more patients to receive the treatment. Racemic ketamine is usually given via an intravenous infusion, whereas Esketamine is given via nasal spray, making it easier to administer. Esketamine has been effective when combined with an oral antidepressant such as Prozac. In one study, 70 percent of the patients with TRD improved on Esketamine compared with the placebo. Following this powerful result, the FDA approved Esketamine for major depression, making it the first new drug approved for major depression in fifty years. Clinical development of ketamine treatment faces many obstacles, primarily because its patent has expired and it therefore receives limited attention from pharmaceutical companies. Combining other medications with a single dose of ketamine can significantly affect outcomes. Trials of Esketamine reported rapid antidepressant effects in patients with treatment-resistant depression in conjunction with an oral antidepressant. One group was given intranasal Esketamine twice weekly for four weeks, together with other antidepressants. Post-administration, they showed reduced depression scores and a significant improvement in suicidal ideation scores after four hours, with a numerical improvement after twenty-four hours. A third of the patients had a resolution of suicidal ideation twenty-four hours after the first dose of Esketamine. Studies using Esketamine for suicidal ideation are ongoing, but the jury is still out on whether it is as strong as traditional ketamine infusions.

Ketamine Administration in the Emergency Department

Emergency departments (ED) are routinely filled with patients with mental illness: suicidal ideations, severe depression, bipolar disorder, mania, and schizophrenia. In the US, there are 400,000 ED admissions annually for suicidal behavior that do not receive timely relief.[22] The rapidity of ketamine's antidepressant effects has sparked great interest in preventing and treating suicide in the ED and acute care settings. In psychiatry, a suicidal patient in the ED is called a "warm hand-off" because the first month after discharge from the hospital or ED is the period for the greatest risk of death by suicide. Ketamine could offer vital support during this vulnerable period, making it an attractive candidate for securing the safety of patients who are at imminent risk of death by suicide.

In an interview with Dr. Thomas Insel, author of the book *Healing: Our Path from Mental Illness to Mental Health*, Insel vocalizes his belief that the real benefit of using ketamine in suicidal patients will be in the ED.[23] "By 2025, we will give ketamine to patients primarily in the emergency departments and less in outpatient clinics," he says. The challenge, for now, is convincing insurance companies and hospitals to adopt new policies and cover the cost of ketamine administration. Dr. Insel explains as we become more adept at diagnosing who is most at risk of suicide, we will naturally move towards using a fast-acting medication like ketamine in emergency departments. It is disturbing that most people who take their lives have touched the mental health care system but have not been targeted for prevention.

"For now, we don't know how to assess risk or who is going to kill themselves in the next twenty-four hours," Dr. Insel says. Ketamine is frequently used in emergency departments to sedate children and adults for procedures; it would be an easy transition for ED doctors to start using ketamine for mental-health emergencies such as suicidal ideation.

Using ketamine to reduce suicidal ideation is gaining acceptance among ED physicians and other acute-care facilities.[24] One ED physician in Los

Angeles described giving a patient sedation for a dislocated ankle. After the procedure, the patient remarked that she saw her mother who passed away sixty years ago and that she felt at peace. The patient thanked the ED physician afterwards.

If a person in the ED for severe depression responds to ketamine, suicidal ideation can be rapidly reduced, possibly avoiding hospital admission. We could safely send the patient home and schedule follow-up care with a mental health professional, similar to what we do for chest pain. Ketamine was given to patients in the emergency department and their symptoms diminished rapidly and significantly within forty minutes, with no evidence of recurrence after a ten-day follow-up.[25] Instead of requiring hospitalization, patients can be cared for in less-restrictive settings and maintain their usual support networks. Being in a hospital is not a deterrent to suicide. We can also use ketamine in inpatient wards, creating a bridge until more extensive help can be mobilized. Ketamine should be seen as a starting point for intensive treatment, not as the singular answer. Currently, ketamine is not routinely used in the ED for patients suffering from suicidal ideation or severe depression due to insurance companies denying coverage. Training the workforce is necessary and expensive but putting the pieces together will reduce risk and save lives. Imagine if Dr. Breen had been offered a medication like ketamine to suppress her suicidal ideation. We will never know, but based on the research, ketamine might have stopped her suicidal ideation, potentially giving her the precious time needed to seek further help. Research is ongoing and hopefully twenty-first-century medicine will evolve, making ketamine available for anyone who needs it.

Postpartum Depression and Ketamine

There is possibly no higher calling in life than to bring a child into the world. Sadly, mothers can become depressed during and after pregnancy and may want to end their life. Similar to a child taking their own life, the suicide of a new mother is shocking and throws a grenade into the family structure. Suicide is a leading cause of death among new mothers.[26] Postpartum depression (PPD) and suicide is the silent health crisis seldom spoken about.[27, 28] PPD suicide usually occurs after childbirth and at any time during the first year. It is estimated PPD occurs in approximately 10–20 percent of mothers, irrespective of culture or race. In the US, nearly 24,000 mothers are at risk of suicide yearly. Suicide during pregnancy or the postpartum period is underreported. A recent study found an increase in suicide attempts during pregnancy and after childbirth, nearly tripling over the past decade.[29]

Postpartum depression severely impairs maternal quality of life and accounts for 20 percent of postpartum suicides. We have no effective preventive treatment or detection methods for PPD. Untreated mental health conditions put mothers and their children at higher risk for adverse health outcomes, including preterm birth and maternal suicide.

Ketamine may have a role in treating PPD and possibly preventing suicide. We know it's safe for mothers because it has been used for decades as an anesthetic during childbirth. In fact, ketamine is one of the very few drugs approved for anesthesia induction in cesarean sections. A study where ketamine was given during childbirth showed a significant improvement in postpartum psychiatric disorders and decreased antenatal depression and suicidal ideation.[30] This study supported the idea that ketamine can prevent postpartum psychiatric disorders. One way ketamine may contribute to a mother's well-being is that it affects the glutamate pathway and increases serotonin and melatonin levels. Together, these findings suggest the increased PPD risk of antenatal depression, moderate stress, and suicidal ideation may be relieved by ketamine. An interesting side note is a new study from Columbia University linking general anesthesia to PPD. A body of research has shown that, compared with regional anesthesia, general anesthesia is linked to an increased risk for PPD after cesarean section.[31] The report's authors believe PPD results from the consequences of general anesthesia, where the patient is unconscious, which delays the first skin-to-skin contact between the mother and child, delaying the first breastfeeding attempt.

Chronic Neuropathic Pain and Ketamine

Neuropathic pain is difficult to treat and requires multiple medications, including narcotics.[32] Hyperalgesia happens when your body's pain receptors are too sensitive, causing pain to feel much more intense than it should; it is triggered when pain-sensing nerves are damaged or severed. Researchers think psychedelics might disrupt these pain connections that become ingrained in the brain. There is research showing ketamine can help treat phantom limb pain that is experienced following the amputation of a limb[33] and there are reports of phantom limb pain completely subsiding after using psychedelics and therapy. A multidisciplinary mind, body, and spirit approach is needed to help these patients. Ketamine allows the patient to remember what it was like to be pain-free. It is an invaluable adjunct medication for treating pain as it decreases the necessity for opioid medications; this is useful in chronic pain treatment and is sometimes life-saving. People with chronic neuropathic pain often have refractory depression, and increasingly, ketamine has been used in both children and adults to treat chronic refractory pain, especially with severe depression.

* * * *

Case Study: Nurse Practitioner with Neuropathic Pain

This nurse practitioner had a chronic pain condition called trigeminal neuralgia resulting from a viral infection. Trigeminal neuralgia is a painful condition that causes intense stabbing sensations similar to an electric shock on one side of the face. It can be so painful that trigeminal neuralgia has been nicknamed the "suicide disease." The cause is most often due to irritation of the trigeminal nerves in the face area resulting from trauma or past infection, or sometimes it starts for no known reason. The pain intensity is so severe that the terms "excruciating" and "incomprehensible" are often used to describe it.

This nurse tried standard therapy for years, including anticonvulsants, physical therapy, and antidepressants. Being on his medications caused him to become disabled, and he could no longer work. His disability caused him to have refractory depression, which eventually became paralyzing. After years of pain, disability, and suffering, his neurologist suggested a lidocaine infusion, which helped intermittently. He was then offered a ketamine infusion for forty-eight hours in the hospital. He described it as a transformative experience and remarked it was the first time in over six years that he could remember what it was like not to feel pain. The ketamine infusion also lifted his depression. He could live normally and return to work with further treatment, even though he was not 100 percent cured.

Source: Shrink Rap Radio Podcast #725. www.shrinkrapradio.com

* * * *

Neurological Basis of How Ketamine Stops Suicide

After nearly half a century, ketamine still occupies a unique corner in the medical armamentarium of physicians treating pain, depression, and suicidality. Yet how ketamine works against suicide and depression is unclear, and the biochemical processes involved in depression go well beyond the monoamine hypothesis, which has dominated psychiatric research for over fifty years. We know ketamine works as a psychedelic, hypnotic, analgesic, and antidepressant. Ketamine affects various cellular functions, including genes, neurotransmitters, hormones, cytokines, and receptors. Some of ketamine's mechanisms may be the increase in glutamate levels, decreasing brain inflammatory molecules, activating proteins like brain-derived neurotrophic factor (BDNF) and mTOR, and inducing neuroplasticity.[34, 35]

The term neuroplasticity was coined in the 1900s. Before then, the adult brain was thought to be a nonrenewable organ, meaning once your brain cells are formed in adulthood, they are finite and cannot be changed or grow back. We now know this isn't true. One leading theory suggests medications like ketamine stimulate the growth of connections between neurons (i.e., neuroplasticity). There are billions of pathways in our brains resembling roads. Some of these roads are more traveled than others. For example, our habits are well-established neural pathways, but as we do new things, we create new pathways in our brains. This is the essence of neuroplasticity. Ketamine increases the functional connectivity in brain circuits, which helps explain its rapid anti-depressive effects.

Scientists always knew children's brains were constantly growing and changing. At birth, an infant's brain has around 7,500 neuronal connections, and this doubles by two years of age. Today, we know that new brain cells and pathways are formed even in old age. We already use medications and chemicals to change how our brains work, and psychology has shown our thought patterns can cause significant changes to our brain structure and function. Enhancing neuroplasticity in adults can result from new environments, new learning, focused cognitive training, physical activity, fasting, restorative sleep, and psychoactive agents such as ketamine and psilocybin.[36, 37] Both pre-clinical and clinical studies show that ketamine reconfigures disrupted prefrontal connectivity, restoring normal metabolic equilibrium, which is referred to as homeostasis by scientists. Brain circuits change in many parts of the brain, including the anterior cingulate cortex, prefrontal cortex, and hippocampus. Abnormalities in these areas, especially the prefrontal cortex and cingulate cortex, have been consistently reported in patients with a history of suicidal ideation.[38] Therefore, ketamine's anti-suicidal action might be related to its ability to restore impaired brain connectivity through neuroplasticity.

Measuring the strength of connections between different brain areas affected by depression is a recent phenomenon. This is important because the increased neuronal conductivity is thought to relieve depression. Traditional antidepressants focus on two neurotransmitters in the brain: serotonin and norepinephrine. An imbalance of these two neurotransmitters was thought to cause depression, and antidepressants restored the balance of these chemicals. However, it was recently found that these chemical changes in the brain occurred quickly after taking antidepressants. It was then surmised antidepressants likely work by increasing the number of new nerve cells and pathways formed in specific brain areas. Psychotherapy, exercise, and ECT[39] are also thought to work in this manner.

Ketamine changes the balance between the neurotransmitters glutamate and GABA. Alcohol is another drug that affects both of these neurotransmitters. Ketamine increases glutamate in the brain by blocking the NMDA receptor and increases communication among existing neurons by creating new connections and enhancing brain circuit activity. Recent research has revealed that ketamine administration in rats[40] and monkeys leads to increased growth and function in the brain, specifically in the dendritic spine synapses in the prefrontal cortex. Glutamate is essential for normal brain functioning, and its levels must be tightly regulated. It is an excitatory messenger and is the workhorse of the brain. It turns on neurons, triggering an electrical impulse. Glutamate is why you can still ride a bike years after you first learned. Eighty percent of large cells in the higher brain release glutamate as their neurotransmitter. Smaller brain cells balance glutamate by releasing the inhibitory neurotransmitter GABA, which quiets brain activity. These excitatory and inhibitory molecules are the most common and important in the brain. Abnormalities in glutamate function disrupt nerve health and communication and, in extreme cases, may lead to nerve cell death. Abnormal levels of glutamate cause many negative symptoms, including pain amplification, anxiety, restlessness, and even seizures. When ketamine binds to the NMDA receptors, it increases the amount of glutamate and neuro-synaptic transmission, thus increasing neuroplasticity.

In the 1990s, through fMRI studies, researchers discovered ketamine causes glutamate release in the PFC and hippocampus.[41] Glutamate then activates another receptor called the AMP-activated protein kinase (AMPK) receptor. Together, the initial blockade of NMDA receptors and the activation of AMPK receptors cause the release of other molecules that help neurons communicate via new pathways. This process likely affects mood, thought patterns, and cognition. Ketamine also has concomitant effects on many systems in the brain—the opioid, dopamine, serotonin, cannabinoid, nitric oxide, noradrenaline, sigma, GABA, and acetylcholine systems. These are all different brain messenger molecules.

The role of the opioid system has recently caught the scientific community's attention, partly because increased suicide rates are linked to the current opioid crisis.[42] The neuropathic pain mechanism differs from other pain types, and ketamine blocks the N-Methyl D-Aspartate (NMDA) receptors involved with neuropathic pain. Since ketamine regulates NMDA receptors, we believe it influences the opiate system as well. In addition, NMDA receptors are involved in the development of opioid tolerance. The opioid system takes part in pain processing, and its involvement in ketamine analgesia has been shown in animal and genetic studies. Adverse experiences like childhood abuse have resulted in epigenetic changes in the opioid system. It is well known that the opioid system is involved in reward, pleasure-seeking, and decision-making systems, and these systems are highly impaired in suicidal behavior.

Interestingly, naltrexone, an opioid receptor partial agonist, has been associated with a decrease in suicidal ideation. Researchers gave TRD patients naltrexone and ketamine[43] and the results showed that ketamine with the addition of naltrexone profoundly attenuated the antidepressant effect. It has been proposed that ketamine alters conscious pain perception. Human studies have shown that a single sub-anesthetic dose of ketamine selectively improves the effective component of pain. These findings are relevant, as suicidality is strongly associated with physical and psychological pain.

Over the years, several studies have corroborated the above results, refining and perfecting our knowledge of the intra-neural underpinnings of the antidepressant action of ketamine and other drugs. Depression is a disease of disconnection at many levels. We associate depression and chronic insomnia with neuronal death and damage. Ketamine, through its action on the glutamate system, induces the quality and quantity of neuronal connections, thus improving the function of critical brain circuits. This allows people to deal more effectively with their problems after receiving medications like ketamine. Many pharmacological treatments are developing that help recovery from depression and suicidal behaviors by encouraging neuroplasticity. Some of these include psilocybin, stem cells, changing gene expression, cellular proliferation, and regulating inflammation and the immune system.

Brain-derived Neurotrophic Factor (BDNF), mTOR, and Ketamine

Healthy brain function depends on having the correct amount of the protein BDNF in the right place and at the right time. Animals and people with depression and suicidal behaviors have low levels of BDNF.[44] Decreased BDNF may predispose to neuronal degeneration, atrophy, and decreased dendritic numbers, leading to low synaptic activity and the clinical symptoms of depression. Brain tissue samples from suicide victims often contain abnormal levels of BDNF. People with severe COVID-19 infections also have low BDNF levels. BDNF is intimately involved in shaping neuronal synapses during brain development and throughout life.

Ketamine increases mTOR and BDNF in the prefrontal cortex and hippocampus.[45] Chronic stress is thought to result in a loss of BDNF-producing brain cells, which leads to reversible structural changes manifested by a loss of connections and nerve cell atrophy.[46] Increasing BDNF levels gives rise to new neuronal connections, branches, and synapses. Intravenous administration of BDNF has a rapid antidepressant effect in animals. Interestingly, in animal models of maternal deprivation, ketamine reverses depressive behaviors after a single dose.[47] They also showed ketamine protects the brain from oxidative stress-induced brain damage by decreasing inflammation.[48] Given ketamine's extensive effects on neuroplasticity and its normalizing effect on the hypothalamic-pituitary axis, ketamine may be helpful in patients with a stress response to suicidal ideation.

Brain-derived neurotrophic factor is a protein that is encoded by the BDNF gene. BDNF is a member of the neurotrophic family of growth factors, discovered in 1980 in swine brains.[49] BDNF acts on specific neurons in the central nervous system and helps to support the survival of existing neurons, encouraging the growth and differentiation of new neurons and synapses. BDNF itself is important for long-term memory. Proteins such as BDNF help stimulate and control brain plasticity. Mice born without the ability to make BDNF suffer developmental effects and die soon after birth, suggesting that BDNF plays a vital role in normal neural development. BDNF initiates synapse formation through its effects on brain-receptor activity and supports the regular everyday signaling necessary for stable memory function. Physical exercise markedly increases BDNF in the human brain, a phenomenon partly responsible for exercise-induced neurogenesis and improvements in cognitive function. BDNF expression is significantly enhanced by the environment. Many studies show links between decreased levels of BDNF in conditions such as depression, schizophrenia, obsessive-compulsive disorder, Alzheimer's disease, Huntington's disease, dementia, anorexia nervosa, and suicidal ideation.[50] BDNF levels are highly regulated throughout the lifetime, both in early development stages and in later stages of life. For example, BDNF appears critical for morphological development in specific brain structures, controlling behavioral processes like learning and motor-skills development. Studies of aging human brains have found that hippocampal volume decreases with decreasing plasma levels of BDNF, partially explaining the cognitive decline that occurs during aging. In addition, BDNF is a critical mediator of vulnerability to stress and stress-related disorders, such as PTSD. Given the reduction in BDNF levels in people with various addictions, this seems a plausible mechanism for ketamine to have an anti-addictive effect.

The mTOR protein modulates several functions, such as neuronal cell activity, metabolism, cell proliferation, death, and protein synthesis. Depressed patients have low activity of mTOR and decreased stimulation of neurons, causing depression. Ketamine rapidly activates the mTOR pathway in the prefrontal cortex, increasing intracellular protein synthesis and cell signaling.[51] Many physiological processes, such as memory formation and neuronal activity, depend on mTOR.

Inflammation, Suicide, and Ketamine

Brain inflammation and suicide are strongly linked. Inflammatory molecules called cytokines, interleukins (IL), and tumor necrosis factor (TNF) are increased in suicidal patients, especially those with diabetes and obesity. These same inflammatory molecules are present in severe COVID-19 infections. However, the mechanisms explaining the anti-suicidal effect of ketamine are unclear. Current evidence points, in part, to the anti-inflammatory effect of ketamine. The causal relationship connecting depression, suicide, and inflammation was discovered in autopsy studies. For example, autopsies of suicide victims showed brain microglial activation consistent with brain inflammation. Another study showed increased levels of IL-6 in the cerebrospinal fluid of suicidal victims. Inflammation leads to the production of molecules that bind to NMDA receptors, and ketamine explicitly blocks the NMDA receptors. It has shown that hippocampal upregulation of inflammatory markers such as IL, TNF, and kyeneurin can all be affected by administering a sub-anesthetic dose of ketamine.[52, 53]

Low-dose naltrexone is an opioid receptor blocker used to treat pain and inflammation in these disorders. Ketamine, given with naltrexone, appears to reduce the production of tumor necrosis factors and interleukins. Ketamine and naltrexone have strong safety records in humans, are inexpensive, and are well tolerated.

Traumatic brain injury also results in brain inflammation. Ketamine is neuroprotective against brain damage from head trauma, strokes, heart attacks, seizures, low oxygen levels (hypoxia), and low blood sugar (hypoglycemia) levels.[54] An intriguing use of ketamine is in the context of chemical warfare. Ketamine may have a role in neuroprotection and reducing neuroinflammation induced by nerve agents such as sarin nerve gas and soman.[55]

Our diet and lifestyles can also cause high levels of brain inflammation. Recent evidence suggests that adopting a non-processed and low-carbohydrate diet can improve symptoms of depression, schizophrenia, and even suicide. Excess consumption of processed carbohydrates and vegetable oils leads to chronic inflammation and excess glutamate in the brain. In Dr. Kate Shanahan's book *Deep Nutrition* she details the harmful effects of processed vegetable oils on the brain.[56] It is arguable that vegetable oils are not meant for human consumption. Excess sugars are responsible for increased inflammation in the modern age. For example, in the 1700s, humans consumed about four pounds of sugar annually. In the 1800s, this increased to over 20 pounds. In the 1900s and into the industrial age, sugar consumption skyrocketed to over 100 pounds per year. Consider that the human body maintains blood sugar levels equivalent to 1 to 2 teaspoons of sugar (75mg/dl or 4mmol). When constantly exposing our bodies to sugar, the body reacts by producing inflammatory factors. Years of chronic sugar exposure causes our bodies to become intolerant to sugar or carbohydrates. The body's response to this excess sugar in the blood is energy storage. In humans, energy is stored in fat cells and causes deregulated energy production and inflammation, leading to brain fog. This is the common link between human obesity and inflammation.

Ketamine is effective for treatment-resistant depression (TRD). It is important to understand the difference between depression and TRD. Imagine battling symptoms of sadness, sleep disturbance, low energy, and thoughts of death or suicide lasting two or more weeks. This is the definition of depression. Now imagine being depressed and trying several medications and therapies—only to discover that none work. This is treatment-resistant depression. Recall that Australian physicians showed that a sub-anesthetic dose of ketamine combined with CBT improved the symptoms of TRD.[57, 58] Some of these patients were on several medications and underwent ECT for several years with no real improvement.[59] Some studies even showed that the effects of ketamine infusions lasted up to six months. In 2012, ketamine research around the world showed a decrease in suicidal ideation in patients; Europe, America, Macao, Israel, Iran, China, and many others demonstrated that ketamine is well tolerated in all ages independent of the method it is administered (oral, intranasal, subcutaneous, intramuscular, or intravenous).

The longer a person is in a state of severe depression and expressing suicidal behavior, the greater the risk of injury and death. A mental disorder, no matter the diagnosis (ADD, depression, bipolar, etc.), will, on average, decrease a person's lifespan by one-third.[60, 61] Because of the high suicide rates and the known relationship between suicidal ideation and attempts leading to death, effective suicide interventions are a national priority. The prospect of averting suicide, preserving life, reducing patient suffering, and saving lives via a rapid reduction in suicidality has substantial public health benefits. We also need to train more primary care physicians to recognize and treat suicidal ideation.

CHAPTER NINE

The Psychedelic Experience and Ketamine Safety

"Psychedelics are to the study of the mind what the microscope is to biology and the telescope is to astronomy."

—*Stanislav Grof*

The therapeutic potential of psychedelics has sparked widespread interest. As we have shown, psychedelic therapy can reverse the debilitating effects of depression, addiction, anxiety, eating disorders, PTSD, and suicidal ideation.

The rapid popularization of these drugs culminated in the prohibition of human studies in the 1960s. We must not forget the lessons of why psychedelics fell out of favor. Many historians point to Timothy Leary, a Harvard researcher who performed academic research on psychedelics.[1,2] However, Leary soon abandoned clinical protocols and began distributing LSD and psilocybin to students and friends. Harvard fired Leary in 1963 when his informal LSD dispensary attracted too much controversy. He continued his research at other institutions and started lecturing across the country, earning the reputation as the "pied piper of LSD" and cultivating the media with sayings like "turn on, tune in, and drop out." Many blame the federal ban on psychedelics at least partly on the role of people like Leary and others, causing anarchy and moral panic. The problem with Leary's approach is that it polluted the potential of psychedelics becoming something better, like a means of treating severe mental illness.

Sixty years later, psychedelic research has returned. Today, despite the laws surrounding psychedelics, over 30 million Americans have tried ayahuasca, LSD, psilocybin, and mescaline in their lifetimes; this inevitably includes many of our lawmakers in Washington, DC. Publications from authors like Michael Pollan (*How to Change Your Mind*)[3] and movements like the Project on Psychedelics Law and Regulation (POPLAR) and US congressman Earl Blumenauer (D-OR) have led to the legalization of some psychedelics; for example, psilocybin in Oregon.[4] This movement could not have come at a more critical time with the mental health crisis. Today, ketamine is the only legal psychedelic available to us with a prescription.

In any enterprise of this sort, it goes without saying that legalization of psychedelics will follow medicalization. Psychedelics go back thousands of years, from ancient Meso-American societies to the ancient Greeks. In those cultures, psychedelics were treated with enormous respect; religious rites grew around them, and psychedelics were controlled by elders and used in rituals. The American Indians used psychedelics in their churches, and today South American shamans guide hundreds through ayahuasca ceremonies.

Psychologist Jordan Peterson ironically once held the same position at Harvard University as Timothy Leary. News articles have even stated that he is "the Leary of this generation." Peterson advocates for psychedelics and psychedelic research, even using them himself. He modified Leary's message to read, "Tune in. Turn on. Grow up," emphasizing that anarchy has to be bound and cognizant to become a higher virtue.[5] That phrasing possibly would have saved us a lot of trouble in bringing psychedelics to a place where they can be used to save lives.

What Is a Psychedelic Experience?

The psychedelic experience is a direct, embodied experience of the mind, body, and spirit; the experience sets the foundation for profoundly introspective regard of the brain and nervous system.[6] Psychedelics have been used for thousands of years, as evidenced by murals found in African,

North American, and European caves dating back more than 5,000 years.[7] *Homo erectus* inevitably encountered and likely ingested psychedelic plants throughout their evolutionary history. North American Indians definitely used psychedelics for thousands of years.

British psychiatrist Humphrey Osmond first coined the term "psychedelic" in 1957; it is derived from the Greek words ψυχή (psyche, "soul, mind") and δηλοῦν (deloun, "to manifest"), hence the term "mind manifesting."[8, 9] Used wisely, sacred plants and psychedelic drugs can offer an opportunity for a deep remedial healing experience, one that repairs despair and annihilates hopelessness with the most meaningful experiences possible. There are several identified dimensions of a mystical experience to include (1) sacredness, (2) noetic quality, (3) deeply felt positive mood, (4) ineffability, (5) paradoxical, and (6) transcendence of time and space.[10]

The hallmarks of a psychedelic experience are very similar to dreams: the third-person perspective, ego-dissolution, higher-order reality, novel insights, and timelessness.

The third-person perspective often brings about a sense of looking back at yourself and your psyche from a detached observation post.

Ego-dissolution is a distance trait of the experience that gives the sense of separation from the self.

Higher-order reality is a sense of "true reality" or a "more real" reality than what is usually available in ordinary consciousness. Some describe it as a feeling of being a "reality hallucination."

Novel insights refer to novel experiences, emotions, insights, revelations, or connections that were not previously understood, known, or embodied as reality.

Timelessness is a manifestation of the experience taking place outside of time. Many describe the notion that time is lost or not present.

As mentioned in an earlier chapter, the psychedelic experience is not strictly limited to a class of compounds or dependent upon the ingestion of a specific substance. Perhaps life itself can be classified as psychedelic under these terms. If you have experienced a psychedelic treatment or know someone who has, the experience often includes several of these characteristics.

This subjective experience, the experiential reality of the ketamine experience, is the strongest argument in favor of classifying ketamine as a psychedelic medicine.[11]

How Psychedelics Work

Sometimes referred to as a reality hallucination, psychedelics temporarily disable the default mode network (DMN).[12] This neural framework constructs our minds and the brain creates some model of reality. Under normal circumstances, the brain filters information from the external world through our sensory neural interface. Most of what we experience never makes it into the brain, and the brain does this so we can cope. We don't reside in "reality" because it would be too overwhelming. What we experience is a schematic or a model of reality that is much less information-dense than the reality of the self. In other words, there are many things we experience that are unimportant and are extraneous to our construction of this model of reality.

We're usually enmeshed inside this DMN framework, which may be helpful for everyday life. To understand why psychedelics successfully treat people with profound depression, we need to know what depression does to people. Depression locks people into a very narrow framework; psychedelics seem to break that lock, allowing openness and new thoughts to enter. The core of the therapeutic promise of psychedelics is they let you step out of this DMN and temporarily look at it as though you know you're separated. It helps give you insights into your existential situation. It enables you to look at trauma, addiction, or depression from a different perspective, one that is usually unattainable. Psychedelics temporarily disable those gating mechanisms. In a sense, they throw the gates wide open and flood you with information that usually is not accessible. This can be beneficial from a therapeutic angle. Our reality model is dysfunctional when you have an addiction, suicidality, depression, and PTSD; psychedelics let you reengineer it in a certain way. The therapeutic effect of psychedelics is reflected on the neurological level because ketamine, psilocybin, and other psychedelics produce changes in neural architecture and connectivity (neuroplasticity).

When you disrupt the DMN, the brain is resilient and always tends toward equilibrium. It's similar to what happens when you reboot or reset your computer and it works more efficiently because you purged all the built-up sludge. People are excited about psychedelics from a therapeutic standpoint because of the ability to disable and reconstruct the DMN more functionally.

Memories have a powerful impact on our bodies. Suppose you have an old memory of a traumatic event that continues to haunt you. When that memory is triggered, the stress reaction from your body is as if the traumatic event were occurring again. The same stress hormones are secreted as if you were actually experiencing the traumatic event. Psychologically, it is an unconscious alarm system causing you to fall into the same pitfalls, called the DMN. This is so significant that people even have heart attacks and strokes from memories.

Our bodies remember stories and are triggered by them more powerfully than words. For example, I often recall 9/11 mainly because I lived it much differently than most. After the Twin Towers had fallen and the skies fell silent, I returned home from the hospital and received a call from my brother that my mother was in the emergency room with chest pain. She had a history of cardiac problems. I thought, at worst, it could be a heart attack, and she would receive treatment at the hospital, but most likely, it was heartburn. I called the emergency room and asked to be connected to the emergency room doctor taking care of my mother. The doctor got on the phone and asked me what kind of doctor I was. I told him that I was an anesthesiologist. He then explained that the news was not good and proceeded to tell me that the medical team was trying to resuscitate my mom as she was in pulseless ventricular tachycardia and thus far they had been unsuccessful. Practically no one survives this lethal arrhythmia.

My heart sank to the ground. I calmly told the doctor to please have the nurses put my family in a separate room, and I respectfully thanked him for his help. I hung up the phone knowing my mom had died and dropped to my knees as I had never done before. That visceral feeling arises in my gut whenever I think about the story. Psychedelics can never block the memory; instead, they make it comfortable enough to relive it with more perspective.

Combine this with proper therapy, and there's a chance the trauma can be reduced close to zero. This is the power of owning your past.

If you run from the trauma, it becomes something bigger than you, and then you feel forced to hide, which is how anxiety manifests itself. It's how we lose sleep. And the more you run from the trauma, the more your body thinks it's winning the race and the more it reinforces the psychological and physiological ailments. It is not always best to face your traumas head-on, but this is why we have community, family, mental health professionals, and psychedelics. Likewise, this is often why young people join gangs, the army, and sports clubs—to be a part of a tribe to sort out their issues. It's helpful to break these traumas into smaller steps and start somewhere specific.

While on psychedelics, you sometimes have a feeling, or you get a definite sense, that you are in a place where people say it seems more real than real.[13] There are entities, or what's perceived as entities, and you're in communication with them, and "they" are very interested in communicating and transmitting the information. After a psychedelic experience, you will be more open-minded, open to options. As Dr. Wolfson says, "you never return quite the same."[14]

Psychedelics continue to teach us how little we know, which is a valuable reminder of our ignorance about the universe or the reality of the way things are. In that sense, psychedelics are instrumental in reminding us that we have only a minuscule portion of it figured out. There's an infinitude of reality beyond that, of which we know nothing; thus, scientists should be humble and always remember we don't know everything.

Psychedelics allow talk therapy to be more effective and less painful. One reason is that psychedelics wash away the ego, creating a safe environment to think about the traumas causing the pathologic stress reactions in the first place. Dr. Karl Friston mentioned on Dr. Jordan Peterson's *Daily Wire Podcast* that neuroticism could be defined as excess chaos or entropy between the person and achieving a balanced state. Psychedelics allow a person to move forward towards a shared goal and decrease the chaos or entropy between getting to that goal.[15] People with mental illness ignore logic simply by suppressing the importance of potential gain or reward. The psyche must become more flexible and adaptable for someone to reach higher levels.[16] This requires a person to become higher on the openness trait. Psychedelics can result in increases in openness even after a single dose.[17, 18] Open people are more creative, thus giving people more play in higher-order conceptualizations. An excellent way to think about it is that if you're more open, there's more play in the system. That's the motivation behind using psychedelics, for example, in end-of-life care.

Psychedelics help with creativity. The effect of a psychedelic experience is so robust that a single mystical experience induced by psilocybin produces about a one-standard-deviation increase in trait openness and creativity that never goes away;[19, 20] ketamine produces similar results.[21] Psychedelics open the barriers between adjacent categories in a person's mind, which thus become more permeable. So then, as information propagates up, there's more play in the systems because the category boundaries have become wider per se. This increases the probability that you'd get some real positives out of the experience, which is what creative people always do. People who take psychedelics mention that ideas become connected in imperceivable ways and produce more flexibility in the system. Neurotic people have limited amounts of flexibility in their conceptual systems.

The past has to die for the future to be realized—one must have the ability to change their mind regarding the past or old concepts. In a sense, we have to die in many situations.[22] Psychotherapy uses psychedelics to rearrange the hierarchy, dissolve barriers, and then rebuild or explore other options. Therapy is about breaking down previous beliefs, allowing them to disintegrate, forgetting what you learned, and rebuilding. Psychedelics allow the rate of transformation to be optimized and allows that optimized process of death, for example, to occur playfully and engagingly instead of being a painful and destructive experience.

There's a metaphor that the walls get higher and higher as you go deeper and deeper because those more fundamental presuppositions alter the amount of entropy released, and it can be so much that it kills you. That's what happens to people with PTSD. For example, military soldiers with PTSD may have some fundamental axiom that is violated, destabilizing them at a deeply fundamental level. It's often a situation where they betray the trust of themselves or others in a malevolent situation, and they become stuck in a particular scenario and cannot redirect. There's some encouraging work on the PTSD front with psychedelics, especially with MDMA.[23] Psychedelic experiences allow one to address the PTSD that ties in with grief. We all go through some trauma in life. If you're psychologically and physiologically compromised, when the trauma hits you, the entropy can destroy you at that point. For example, this might manifest itself when you lose someone close to you when you're not physiologically viable, and that might be enough chaos to do you in.

The Psychedelic Dream Function

A psychedelic experience carries messages rich in symbolic language and quality. Describing what it feels like is challenging to explain. Camila Sanz investigated this topic and published an analysis of subjective reports of dreams of different altered states of consciousness and their relationship to brain physiology.[24, 25]

In psychedelic integration, we have to work with the language of the psyche—the symbolic, mystery, and archetypal layers of our being. As with dreams, the visions, myths, and symbols that spontaneously emerge in expanded states from one's depths are imbued with meaning and express vital psychological information. They carry into consciousness thoughts, intuitions, and feelings that are deeply buried and may not be accessible except through a psychedelic experience or dream state.[26, 27]

The tendency of dreams and psychedelic drugs to induce visionary experiences inspired scientific and cultural development for thousands of years. Both sleep and psychedelics induce profound effects on emotion activation, fear memory extinction, mental imagery, perception, and sense of self and body, and both dreams and psychedelics share neurophysiological features. Psychedelic states may be understood as "experimental dreams." Dreaming is "the purest form of imagination," an involuntary but organized mental act that originates in abstract knowledge and symbolic thinking. Dreams are signaled back to perceptive areas to generate "embodied simulations" of the natural world. Dreaming always induces alterations in the sense of self and body. Self-centered perspective is usually strong and vivid in dreams: the dreamer is inside the scene, taking part in the dream events from a first-person perspective or looking at the events as an external observer.

Classical psychedelics are unique psychoactive drugs whose distinguishing feature is the "capacity reliably to induce states of altered perception, thought, and feeling that are not experienced otherwise except in dreams or at times of religious exaltation." This psychedelic-induced disinhibition leads to an inability to screen out exteroceptive and interoceptive stimuli, which causes a sensory overload of higher-level cortical regions and the formation of hallucinations.

The neuronal mechanisms underlying psychedelic-induced visual mental imagery have been studied using functional magnetic resonance imaging (fMRI). Researchers have found that psychedelics like ayahuasca significantly increased activation in the mental imagery condition within an extended mental imagery network, including early visual areas, the parahippocampal gyrus, the middle temporal cortex, and the frontal cortex.[28] Most importantly, they showed that activation in the primary visual cortex during mental imagery was comparable to activation during perception. Ayahuasca enhances the intensity of voluntary imagery to the same level as a perceived image, lending reality status to inner experiences. There is consistent evidence that psychedelics modulate neural processes related to anxiety and threat, especially in brain regions that are relevant for conditioned fear memory, such as the amygdala, hippocampus, and ACC. Moreover, there is accumulating evidence from animal studies showing that psychedelics may facilitate the extinction of conditioned fear memory by enhancing BDNF-dependent neuroplasticity.

Therefore, psychedelic-induced retrieval of emotional memories, especially contextual information related to fear and anxiety, might facilitate fear extinction via effects on memory modulation and re-consolidation if there is no reinforcement by the unconditioned stimulus. Therefore, it is conceivable that psychedelics might facilitate conditioned fear extinction if the conditioned fear memory is retrieved.

Taken together, although both dreams and psychedelic states share an everyday phenomenological and neurobiological basis, there are also some differences between them, mainly due to more significant perceptual influences from the external environment, clarity of consciousness, and meta-cognitive abilities in psychedelic states compared to REM sleep. There is accumulating evidence that we are not sleeping during dreams.

The many types of dreams that can occur in psychedelic states are pre-cognitive dreams that have arrived from a future point that might inform the dreamer about something yet ahead of him. Apparition dreams are palpable visitation dreams where the person might meet, engage with, or receive a message from a person or persons who have died, whom they may or may not know. They come as psychic allies to offer the dreamer information, guidance, or reassurance. Lucid dreams are dreams where the person feels awake within a dream, able to consciously engage with the dream images and spaces they are immersed in. Disembodied voice dreams are where the person is advised by a voice that exists separately from a body or a voice that might carry. Dreams of deep silence are dreams that land the person in the space of a deep silent void. The silence might be meditative, healing, therapeutic, deadening, or frightening, as a voiceless cry for help. Waking dreams are visions in a hypnagogic or somnambulant state during which the person watches moving images, like in a cinema. Many describe psychedelic dreams as being held and cradled by an archetypal and transpersonal entity, giving psychedelic dreamers a tangible, visceral, and embodied experience of being safely contained.

Psychedelic experiences, like dreams, take form through our lives and need to be understood within the ancestral, biographical, and present-day context of a person's life. When such material is worked through within a therapeutic framework, it can help us develop stability, resilience, and ego strength by assimilating more of our unconscious into consciousness.

The rationale behind this approach was that psychedelics are not pharmacotherapeutic "medications" per se but tools to enhance psychotherapeutic processes via introspective experiences. This therapeutic approach was termed "psycholytic therapy," showing that psychedelics facilitate access to self-relevant processes by reducing cognitive control ("defense mechanisms," in psychodynamic terms) and enhancing mental imagery. One reason this might happen is that ketamine blocks glutamate receptors, and one of the primary neurotransmitters involved in conditioned fear learning is glutamate.

The Ketamine Psychedelic Experience

Ketamine is the one medication where it is legal and acceptable to go to a doctor and be prescribed a psychedelic experience.[29] The goals are to reopen the individual's sensitivity and sensibility and reinstate their humanity and vulnerability to the world. We all carry an emotional armor that restricts expression and the love a person can give to themselves and others. With ketamine, the habitual defenses are removed as consciousness is dissociated from the body.

Most report the experience of ketamine to be pleasant, describing:

"Ketamine filled in my missing piece."

"I feel whole for the first time since the accident 33 years ago."

"The world was brighter."

"A Christmas miracle."

"I was finally standing up straight and experiencing the world."

"It was like it melted my armor (of depression)."

"It was like I was in a biological membrane . . . very pleasurable."

It is essential to establish that ketamine is a medication that acts on our nervous systems—the brain, heart, and gut. The experience of ketamine happens in the mind and body, and everyone's experience is unique. Most patients describe a profound, magical, enlightening, and intense experience from ketamine.

Some patients describe the sensory effects of ketamine as including a visible buzzing, vibrating field around physical objects. Some describe the melting of boundaries of those objects. There may be magnification, diminution, or alteration of color intensity and hue. Colors sometimes generate auditory impressions, a blending of sense information called synesthesia. Likewise, visualization of sounds, as well as unheard rhythms, have been described. Psychedelics may allow users to see and experience things not possible in ordinary reality. In addition, what people may experience with their eyes closed may be superimposed on the outside world when they open their eyes. People often describe detailed geometric shapes or enhanced details of a movement or picture. These "visions" can be extraordinarily complex and may comprise well-formed and recognizable objects like living creatures, machinery, and landscapes. Sounds usually become softer or sometimes painfully harsh. The effects on tactile and gravitational senses are pronounced.

Rapid fluctuation of emotions between joy, anger, passion, hatred, shame, and grandiosity is typical. Other times, a person may feel no emotions at all. Thinking may speed up or slow down. Many people experience new or philosophical insights, especially when the proper forethought and coaching occur through therapy or meditation. Ketamine produces a sense of reality that may feel "more real than real" or like "a cosmic Disneyland." Information arises from novel sources such as clouds, flowers, pictures, and objects.

Psychedelics usually produce a state of increased suggestibility. Many describe an expanded sense of empathy for other people, animals, plants, and objects. Ketamine, when appropriately given, results in a peaceful experience that gives the person a break from reality.

Hamilton Morris, a chemist who hosts the show *Hamilton's Pharmacopeia*, describes ketamine as being similar to phencyclidine (PCP) but much shorter in duration, more of a psychedelic experience, and more sedating.[30] Movement can be difficult, which makes it ironic that ketamine is often taken at dance-rave parties. With higher doses, you recede into yourself and enter a lucid, dreamlike state. The imagery becomes increasingly abstract. Other psychedelics do not have the same effects, and dissociative anesthetics tend to produce more random images.

Who Should Use Ketamine?

There is a wide range of indications for the consideration of ketamine. Most commonly, ketamine is used for people with PTSD, severe depression, TRD, side effects from antidepressants, chronic pain syndromes, substance abuse disorders, OCD, and eating disorders; for self-enlightenment; and for suicide prevention. An interesting use for ketamine is in bipolar disorder with the fear of harm phenotype, which is a disorder that rarely responds to traditional psychiatric drugs.

* * * *

Case Study: James

James is a creative director and enjoys spending time with his wife and kids. However, it wasn't always like this. Despite having a happy childhood, he describes his thoughts as out of control. He describes an overwhelming innate fear, causing him to literally sleep with the cover over his head with just enough room to breathe through his mouth. James describes the fear as akin to crossing a busy freeway. His body temperature was always hot, so that he slept with the windows open in the winter. In his twenties, James saw a doctor who diagnosed him with ADD, so he started taking stimulants. He found himself putting things together and then taking them apart repeatedly, feeling like he was in a massive downward spiral. He had always suffered from mood swings, but now they were becoming rapid and extreme, and his thoughts circled around gruesome scenarios. After finding himself unable to work, James sought help from Dr. Papolos in New York. He was diagnosed with a violent type of bipolar disorder called the fear of harm phenotype. This disorder rarely responds to traditional psychiatric drugs, so James started taking ketamine nasal spray every other day. His response was dramatic. He stopped overheating. On the first day, he turned to his wife and said he felt calm. James started working on his computer again and was able to fully return to work a month later.

Source: NPR—"From Chaos to Calm: a Life Changed by Ketamine," 2018.[31]

* * * *

Some patients report "an unpleasant experience" after taking ketamine, likely because ketamine creates deep insights and openings to the psyche, helping us reestablish connections and honest truths that we may not want to be open to. By opening truths, we are given options to move ahead and explore why we hurt so badly. Ketamine treatments may go awry if conducted while the patient is acutely withdrawing from certain medications and alcohol. Psychologist Jordan Peterson famously described a bad experience with ketamine in the preface of his new book, *Beyond Order: 12 More Rules for Life*. He says, "I ceased using the benzodiazepine entirely in May

2019, trying two doses of ketamine within a week, as suggested by the psychiatrist with whom I consulted. Ketamine, a nonstandard anesthetic/psychedelic, sometimes has overwhelming and sudden positive effects on depression. It produced nothing for me but two ninety-minute trips to hell. I felt to my bones as if I had everything to feel guilty and ashamed about, with nothing gained by my positive experiences." Peterson's "hellish" experiences likely stem from the fact he suffered acute benzodiazepine withdrawal, which can kill a person. There is certainly more to his story, but it's quite possible that Peterson would react differently to ketamine now that he is thankfully recovered from the effects of the benzodiazepines. Hopefully, you can appreciate that ketamine is not for everybody. I met Peterson and prefaced my question about his disdain for ketamine, and then I presented the idea of this book to him. He was exquisitely curious about the subject and politely asked me to send my book to his agent.

To better comprehend why some people may have an unsatisfactory experience with psychedelics like ketamine, it is essential to understand that the psychedelic experience connects us to many experiences. One of those experiences is suffering—deep visceral suffering. A poor experience conceivably stems from the person judging the experience versus just letting it happen. Many people's personalities are developed to help them escape the pain. The other thing that leads to an unpleasant experience is that the person does not have the proper guidance or environment. Psychedelic experiences are often directed by inexperienced guides posing as healers and shamans. This is why it is essential to have legitimate psychological therapy around ketamine or any psychedelic treatment. That being said, there are no "bad experiences" per se. There are only difficult ones whose meaning we have not yet understood and integrated into our lives. The pain, fear, or terror only surfaces because it is already there. Better to be aware of it and revisit it with awareness, strength, and a proper mindset.

The ketamine molecule does not "contain" a psychedelic experience per se; instead, your consciousness delivers the experience. Subjective descriptions of the ketamine experience include a sense of detachment from the body (dissociation), enhancement of insight into reality, and a sense of relaxation or well-being. A sub-anesthetic dose of ketamine is a powerful psychedelic medication that makes it possible to have a conscious experience. It is a journey that usually lasts about an hour. Ketamine gives the person a break from reality, which is one reason it is helpful. Ketamine can have very different effects depending on your expectations and the environmental setting. The desire to use ketamine to blow off steam and relax will generate a different experience than it would for someone seeking to correct a mental illness.

The ketamine experience resembles the plant psychedelics like ayahuasca in South America, DMT, or psilocybin. People have profound psychological and philosophical experiences with ketamine and ayahuasca, and many go on to make profound life changes after the experience, such as disconnecting from dysfunctional relationships, changing from miserable jobs, kick-starting new careers, enrolling in higher education, and more. There are many differences between the psychedelic experiences of ketamine, ayahuasca, or psilocybin. One difference between ketamine and ayahuasca is that people generally describes the ketamine experience as more intense and they do not experience the severe nausea and vomiting associated with the psychedelic plant.

Ketamine filters reality, so one gains an enhanced appreciation for the world outside of categorical, everyday knowledge. With psychedelics, patients have subjective experiences where they feel they have gained new insights into their understanding of reality, as though a curtain has been lifted or a wall removed. This feeling is not a sort of inebriation or intoxication. After being under the influence of ketamine, the world does not appear to fit into verbal labels and categories, and everything seems connected rather than linear.

To put this in perspective, imagine that our brains resemble a communist country like North Korea, which is governed by an authoritarian regime that tries to ensure nobody learns about the outside world through the internet or television. Our brain is similar in how it allows information to enter and leave. Typically, our brains filter out specific thoughts and experiences that do not seem to fit our pattern or template of our quotidian experience. But when a person is experiencing ketamine, the brain realizes thoughts and information are abstract from reality. Consider the example:

You may have an extreme fear of having a needle inserted into your vein. Even if you tell yourself that a tiny needle will save your life, your brain will not accept this information but instead will fixate on how the needle will hurt you. Once that information from the outside world slips in, our brains quickly eradicate that knowledge. Under the influence of a psychedelic like ketamine, our brains filter out reality (the fear of needles in this case), so we can experience a different type of reality in which we each separate our thoughts and try to advance our personal goals. Often, the experience results in the person having less or no fear of needles.

Ketamine and Near-Death Experiences

Near-death experiences (NDEs) sound scary but can be transformative in some people, inducing hopeful changes in spiritual development and worldview.[32, 33] Ketamine-induced NDEs appear to be equivalent to natural NDEs. The psychology of NDEs may be an adaptive mechanism of the mind that alerts a person to the threat of death while the potential tidal wave of fear is kept at bay. This model may apply to situations like falling from a cliff and was developed initially from near-death experiences in mountain climbers. We know one part of the mind can split off or dissociate from another for psychological reasons. The purpose of this may be protection from anxiety so the ego can attend to unfinished business.

The mystical experiences and psychedelic effects of ketamine have been linked not only with positive outcomes in various treatments but also those described as "life-changing" and "spiritually meaningful." The mystical experience of ketamine is important in its therapeutic mechanism. A sense of timelessness and eternity is also often experienced. Ketamine alters the default mode network, decreasing maladaptive, repetitive thoughts. The near-death experience (NDE) is an altered state of being that can be reached in various ways, including through drugs like DMT (dimethyltryptamine) and ketamine. We can reproduce all the features of a classical NDE in some people when ketamine is accurately administered. There are no agreed criteria defining the NDE. Fundamental features include a sense that what is experienced feels real and that what is happening is inexpressible in words. Although there are often feelings of peace, joy, and euphoria, some cases have been frightening and unpleasant. The initial events may sometimes happen at high speed. Some describe being on a roller coaster, while many describe out-of-body experiences. Kenneth Ring, the author of *Life and Death*, classifies the NDE five-stage continuum: feelings of peace, detachment from the body, entering a transitional world of darkness (rapid movement through a long dark tunnel or "the total trip"), emerging into bright light, and entering the light. Ketamine allows some patients to reason that the strange, unexpected intensity and the unfamiliar dimension of their experience mean they must have died. The effects of an NDE can include an enhanced joy in living, reduced fear of death, increased concern for others, reduced levels of anxiety, reduced addiction, improved health, and resolution of various symptoms.

Ketamine has even been said to be neuro-protective in actual near-death situations, meaning it can prevent brain damage from lack of oxygen or blood sugar, which may result from interruption of the blood supply during a heart attack or stroke.[34] Interestingly, patients with severe oxygen depriva-tion during prolonged periods have had profound near-death experiences and, to the doctor's astonishment, sometimes survived the episode with-out impaired brain function. The lack of damage may result from blocking over-excitation, which is also how ketamine acts on the brain. Some who experience an NDE are less likely to suffer brain damage when the blood supply to the brain is impaired. Magnesium also blocks glutamate, protect-ing cells from damage and stopping seizures.

Interestingly, sleep and dreaming involve the glutamate system. Interference with glutamate transmission has dramatic effects. A vivid example is the extensive loss of glutamate-releasing cells in Alzheimer's and, to a lesser extent, schizophrenia. Most large brain cells release glutamate, which also plays a crucial role in intelligence, memory, personality, and the features that make us human. Language, thinking ahead, making tools, and abstract thought are all known examples. Glutamate is also the primary messenger of sensation and perception, and ketamine affects all these areas.

The Safety of Ketamine

Ketamine's tolerability and safety have been demonstrated for over seventy years. Many reports describe patients taking legitimate ketamine consistently for over ten or fifteen years without indications of tolerance, dependence, or addiction.[35, 36] An extensive body of evidence shows the safety of using ketamine in office anesthesia and analgesia in emergency departments, operating rooms, and outpatient pain management clinics.[37] Ketamine is used in small doses to treat depression, and when used for general anesthesia, an anesthesiologist gives ketamine upwards of ten times the dose prescribed for depression. Note that when ketamine is used for general anesthesia, the brain is sent into a chemical coma per se, and ketamine is not an antidepressant at this dose. For most ketamine treatments, a medical professional should be present and prepared to handle any adverse medical situations.

The most common side effects are dizziness, dry mouth, coordination problems, nausea, and tiredness. Other reported experiences include euphoria, feelings of unreality, blurred vision, disorientation, anxiety, and hallucinations. Every one of these side effects is transient, meaning they quickly resolve.[38]

A review of over 70,000 published articles on ketamine highlights its safety.[39, 40] Studies from three different clinical trials of sub-anesthetic, intravenous ketamine administration for major depressive disorders found adverse effects, including dizziness, self-actualization, and drowsiness. Whether these effects are benign or a part of ketamine's actual effects that resulted in therapeutic benefit is a subject of debate. About a third of patients experience mildly elevated heart rate and blood pressure. Some patients will develop anxiety from the dissociative side effects of ketamine. Often, proper coaching and environment minimize these risks.

Many people also report difficulty with balance, minor numbness, muscle weakness, and impaired vision after receiving ketamine. The dose and route of administration can predict the drug's side effects; when the absorption of ketamine is rapid, as by the intravenous, intramuscular, or intranasal routes, the frequency and severity of side effects are greater. When ketamine is given orally, the side effects seem to be less. A calm and positive environment is essential. It is not advisable to watch alien movies like *Men in Black* while experiencing ketamine.

A medical exam should always be performed before giving ketamine. The drug is rarely a problem in otherwise healthy adults. However, ketamine can have different effects on small children and the elderly. Patients with cardiac problems, such as high blood pressure or arrhythmia, require monitoring. Ketamine can cause transient increases in blood pressure and heart rate. This is usually good, as most anesthetics decrease heart rate and blood pressure. Mild heart palpitations may occur but are usually transient. Most anesthetics and sedatives will decrease breathing but ketamine has little effect on the respiratory system. Patients breathe normally while receiving ketamine, especially at the sub-anesthetic dose used in a ketamine clinic.

Ketamine-related bladder problems (cystitis) have been reported, including painful urination, decreased urine flow, and bloody urine. However, nearly all of these have been addicts who often take large recreational doses of street ketamine, upwards of 3 to 10 grams. This is over 1,000 times the typical dose for intravenous ketamine used in a clinic. Furthermore, street ketamine often contains fentanyl and other impurities not found in pharmaceutical-grade ketamine. Bladder problems like cystitis have not been reported as an outcome in any published trials of ketamine.[41] Yet authors writing in psychiatric journals continue to insinuate that all ketamine use can cause cystitis, taking the problem out of context.[42] Many burn units have administered ketamine daily to victims for months at a time to facilitate dressing changes.[43] Overall, ketamine has a low rate of serious side effects. The multiple research trials of thousands of ketamine administrations given by physicians clearly show the potential benefits far outweigh the risks.[44]

* * * *

Case Study: Chemical Engineer (Anonymous)

I have benefited from ketamine infusions to treat chronic major depressive disorder. I credit the doctors for saving my life, but I get annoyed when "experts" complain about the side effects of ketamine. These side effects are far less damaging than the potentially terminal outcome of treatment-resistant depression (TRD) or the impact of TRD on your life, job, and those around you. The potential for addiction to ketamine is always overstated. Infusions start at 0.5 mg/kg, way below the levels used by ketamine abusers and even the levels used by anesthesiologists who administer ketamine daily. I do, however, agree the long-term impact has yet to be evaluated, but I stand by my assertion I'll deal with the complications in the future for life now. Besides, ketamine infusions feel good, and there is plenty of anecdotal evidence that having an out-of-body experience suggests greater efficacy. The worst side effects I've experienced were nausea and vomiting, but Zofran (antiemetic) treats that when given prophylactically.

The saddest part of all this is ketamine costs just a few dollars and relieves major depression almost instantly. Unfortunately, insurers won't offer this treatment, as it is "off label," resulting in huge out-of-pocket costs. Part of the reason no company would fund the testing to approve ketamine for a new use is because there would be no patent-protected profit. So it spurs some research, and Janssen develops a patentable method to prepare a single enantiomer (hardly a simple process) and then gets approval for its use to treat depression when delivered intranasally. I am all for a company making money, but plain old ketamine works by infusion, IM injection, orally, and nasally. However, Janssen's "rack rate" for Esketamine is over twice the cost of the out-of-pocket ketamine infusion (approval trials and development are not cheap, after all). Of course, insurance will pay a fraction of that, but I am guessing the total cost to the insurer, plus your copay, will still be significantly more than a ketamine infusion.

Source: chemistry doctor example taken from C&EN (cen.acs.org)

* * * *

The Addiction Potential of Ketamine

Ketamine and all psychedelics must be treated with respect. Ketamine dependence can happen but is different than being addicted to heroin or alcohol. The main difference is that humans do not experience withdrawal reactions from ketamine, whereas the withdrawal reactions from heroin and alcohol can be life-threatening. However, ketamine addicts will continually make the same poor choices as they do with heroin and alcohol until they are able to break the dependence through help or willpower. Precaution and safety should be considered when using psychedelics in both healthy subjects and patients, given that psychedelics are potent modulators of consciousness states and given that previous history (e.g., Timothy Leary) has shown that the self-enhancing effects of psychedelics might also have adverse long-term effects if not provided within a supervised professional setting. It has been said that Dr. John Lilly used ketamine for many years and could only break the addiction near the end of his life.

Long-term recreational use of ketamine usually involves street ketamine and leads to tolerance, dependence, and addiction about 5 to 10 percent of the time. The highest risk potential is for those with other substance addictions, such as heroin. This seems ironic since ketamine can treat addiction to other drugs. Street ketamine often contains other contaminants and substances, which can contribute to dependency. Still, it remains an uncommon drug used by less than 1 percent of people in the US, according to a study published in the *American Journal of Public Health*.

Edward Domino's article, "Taming the Ketamine Tiger," succinctly tells the story of Marcia Moore and ketamine addiction.[45] In 1978, Moore, a celebrated yoga teacher, met Howard Alltounian, MD, a respected clinical anesthesiologist. They reportedly used ketamine together, fell in love, and were married shortly after. Moore and Alltounian felt they were pioneering a new path to consciousness. Ms. Moore was called the "priestess of the Goddess Ketamine." She took the drug daily and developed a tolerance. Her husband warned her of its dangers. She slept only a few hours each night. She agreed she was wrong about many things and was "going to stay with it until it is tamed." However, Moore could not tame the ketamine tiger, and she disappeared in January 1979. The assumption was that she injected herself with ketamine and froze to death in a forest. Two years later, her skeletal remains were found. Stories like these are thankfully rare.

Ketamine has been demonstrated to be an incredibly safe drug when given appropriately in a proper setting. Overdosing from ketamine is possible, as with any medication. However, all these risks are minimized if taken in a clinic or under physician supervision. Ketamine given in hospitals and clinics is unadulterated and pharmaceutical grade. David Feifel studied 6,000 patient encounters describing just nine cases of addiction attributed to using ketamine in a clinic.[46] Most of these patients had pre-existing addictions. A comprehensive, systematic review of ketamine found no reports of ketamine use or misuse following appropriate treatment with ketamine, nor was there evidence of transition from medical to non-medical ketamine use.[47, 48]

Who Should Not Use Ketamine?

There are very few absolute contraindications to trying ketamine, but certain groups will require more intensive monitoring. Allergies to ketamine are rare, and a recent medical publication cited that four apparent allergic reactions have been reported over the past fifty years.[49] In patients with cardiovascular instability, particularly uncontrolled high blood pressure, ketamine may be safer than alternatives but would require cautious dosing and a high level of supervision. Ketamine causes nausea in some patients, and a subset cannot tolerate the vomiting. The nausea can effectively be treated with an anti-nausea medication, Zofran. A small percentage do not respond to ketamine, even at high intramuscular doses, especially those with rigid personality structures, severe obsessive-compulsive disorder, or other personality disorders. People with difficulty entering a trance state often cannot sustain the benefits they experience from a session. Ketamine should be given cautiously to people with active psychotic disorder (mania). People who ingest massive doses of ketamine over long periods can have a persistent psychosis that is not amenable to currently available treatments. People intoxicated with other substances should not be given ketamine.

In pregnancy, safety is not established.[50] As of 2014, the FDA has not formally assigned ketamine to a pregnancy category. Animal studies at higher-than-human doses failed to reveal evidence of teratogenicity or impairment of fertility; however, there are no controlled data on human pregnancy. Since its safe use in pregnancy and delivery has not been established, the manufacturer recommends ketamine be contraindicated for pregnant women, even though it is regularly administered in obstetric anesthesia. The FDA has not classified ketamine under a pregnancy risk category. Australia's category is B3: "Drugs which have been taken by only a few pregnant women and women of childbearing age, without an increase in the frequency of malformation or other direct or indirect harmful effects on the human fetus having been observed. Animal studies have shown evidence of increased fetal damage, the significance of which is uncertain in humans." Ketamine breastfeeding warnings state: "There is no data on the excretion of ketamine into human milk. But the drugs and lactation database show that ketamine and its metabolites appear in breast milk at very low levels. Ketamine should be undetectable in maternal plasma approximately 11 hours after a dose. Nursing after this time should not expose the infant to significant amounts of the drug." And for closed-angle glaucoma: "There is a minor risk of increased intraocular pressure."[51]

CHAPTER TEN

Ketamine:
The Future and Beyond

"Never let the future disturb you. You will meet it, if you have to, with the same weapons of reason which today arm you against the present."

—*Marcus Aurelius,* Meditations

Ketamine Clinics

Finding a ketamine infusion can be challenging, depending on who is helping you and where you live. The first step is to speak to your doctor, primary care provider, or mental health provider. While your primary care provider will not likely be able to provide ketamine infusion therapy at their office, they can help refer you to a reputable ketamine clinic. At a ketamine infusion center, you will undergo an initial assessment with a doctor to determine if ketamine therapy is right for you. During this assessment, a doctor will review your medical and mental-health histories. Always let the doctor know of any medications that you are taking. There are a few medications that can react with ketamine, such as Lamictal and some benzodiazepines. It is also essential to let your doctor know if you are using anything like marijuana, cocaine, or alcohol because any of these can interfere with the ketamine and create problems. It is best to be upfront, honest, and transparent about your addiction or substance abuse. Addiction will not disqualify you from receiving ketamine treatments. In fact, the treatment may

159

provide added benefits when it comes to dealing with your addiction issues. It would help if you also let your doctor know of any additional conditions you are dealing with, such as chronic pain syndromes, PTSD, OCD, or fibromyalgia.

Once you have received the green light to move forward with ketamine, you can schedule your first treatment. Most treatments are scheduled for thirty to sixty minutes. Someone will need to be with you to drive you home. Short-term side effects include a dissociative state, mild sedation, dizziness, nausea, and vomiting. These side effects are often short-lived and are more likely to occur if you are on multiple substances, such as marijuana or alcohol. The good news is there are no reported long-term side effects reported in humans with pharmaceutical-grade low-dose ketamine.

At most clinics, you will be given ketamine through an intravenous line or intramuscular injection; it can also be delivered via nasal spray, oral lozenges, or sublingual tablets. Ketamine is often dosed based on weight, and there is no standard or "magic dose." Most clinics start with a low dose and continue to adjust until they reach a dosage that effectively treats your symptoms.

During the ketamine experience, you must be sedated and not asleep to receive the benefits. When ketamine is used in doses that cause sleep, patients do not receive the same antidepressant effect. The number of treatments your doctor will recommend will depend on your psychological or physical issues and how your body responds to the ketamine treatments. Many clinics will prescribe three to six treatments to maximize the effects of the ketamine, but the number of treatments can vary widely from person to person. Some people require periodic treatments, while others no longer require ketamine after a single dose.

Ketamine-infusion therapy is a potentially incredible tool if you are struggling with severe depression, but it should only be given under the supervision of a medical professional. Using ketamine without the guidance of a medical doctor is strongly discouraged, unsafe, and even illegal. Street ketamine is often laced with other chemicals and can be harmful. The dissociative state caused by ketamine can put you in danger under the wrong circumstances.

Ketamine is a safe medication under medical supervision. Some clinics prescribe oral ketamine to be taken at home, but only under the supervision of a medical doctor. There are hundreds of ketamine clinics nationwide. Outpatient ketamine clinics also treat chronic pain syndromes such as fibromyalgia, migraines, complex regional pain syndrome, neuropathic pain, and radiculopathy. Many emergency departments are rediscovering the value of using ketamine for patients presenting with suicidal ideation. They also use it for sedation in other procedures like suturing wounds and setting broken bones.

Things to Know Before Going to a Ketamine Clinic

Insurance rarely covers ketamine treatments so they usually must be paid out of pocket and may cost hundreds of US dollars per infusion. The prices are higher in metropolitan areas like New York and Los Angeles and lower in rural areas. The most important consideration in any clinic is patient safety. A physician staffs most clinics; however, in some states, a nurse practitioner or physician assistant (PA) can work independently, and there may be no physician involvement. Several nurse practitioners have opened ketamine clinics, but many have had no inpatient hospital experience, much less critical care or anesthesia experience. These clinics are poorly prepared to handle emergencies. Be sure to ask if a physician is present at the clinic. If you do not feel safe or comfortable in the clinic, go elsewhere. Unexpected medical issues can arise, and the clinic you choose should be able to handle an emergency, such as an airway or cardiac issue.[1]

Ketamine treatments are more effective in conjunction with a mental health provider. Many clinics require a referral from a psychologist or psychiatrist. Always bring your medical records with you. If you are a parent and want your child to be treated with ketamine, most clinics will require a primary care and psychiatry evaluation and referral.

Dr. David Feifel is a board-certified neuropsychiatrist and founder of the Kadima Neuropsychiatric Institute in San Diego, California. He is a professor of psychiatry at the University of California at San Diego. Ten years ago, he opened one of the first ketamine-infusion centers for psychiatric disorders. A prolific author, Dr. Feifel has been at the forefront of using ketamine for mental disorders. He estimates about seven out of ten patients improve their depression after ketamine.[2, 3]

Dr. Joel Friedman has been treating patients for many years in his Hawaii-based clinic. He provides each of his patients with this letter to help them understand the principles of the treatment:

Dr. Friedman's "K" Treatments

Currently, we are experiencing a resurgence of interest in using sub-anesthetic doses of ketamine. We have Yale Medical School largely to thank for this, as they began looking into it as a treatment for suicidal ideation, and now it's used as a treatment for PTSD and depression. Most of us in the medical world know that we have virtually no effective treatment for suicidal patients, yet Yale was finding an immediate effect. This caught my attention, and it was not long after (actually, the very next day after reading the article) a young man presented to my office with suicidal ideation as his chief complaint. He was not expecting a smile from his doctor and asked why I was grinning. I replied, "Funny that you should come today. Yesterday, I would have nothing to offer you. Today, I have a very interesting and hopeful treatment." I explained the details about ketamine and asked if he was interested. "Of course, I am." I asked him to rate his level of suicidal ideation on a scale of 1–10, with a 10 being "pass me the gun." He responded, "nine." Right there, he laid on the examining table, which is more ample than the typical examining table and quite comfortable to stretch out. I gave him headphones to block out ambient noise and an eye pillow to block out light. I then gave him 35 mg of ketamine in his vein as a quick shot. I sat and watched for the next 20 minutes, not knowing what to expect. He was completely still, and his breath became slow and full. Outwardly, not much happened. He slowly came around after 20 minutes and took off the headphones and eyeshades. The first word out of his mouth was, "Wow," which is pretty much everyone's first time reaction. We spoke a bit afterward, but finding words was difficult. It became clear this experience defies description, and this seems fairly universal; I will get to this soon. I asked him to rate his level of suicidal ideation after the ketamine, hoping I miraculously reduced it to a "six." He looked puzzled and responded, "zero." I asked again, thinking he did not understand my question. He repeated, zero. Now, it was my turn to be speechless. Going from a nine to a zero in 20 minutes, in terms of wanting to kill oneself, was, simply put, a miracle. I had never seen or heard of this before, nor had any of my colleagues. I knew we were onto something very special and I have been doing ketamine sessions ever since for conditions which include depression, PTSD, bipolar illness, and anxiety. The only mental conditions in which I will not use ketamine are schizophrenia and borderline personality disorder. This is not a treatment for anyone who does not have a decent grip on reality. I screen every patient and will not use ketamine if I am uncomfortable. The results have been close to universally beneficial. The level of benefit ranges from mild to life changing. Sometimes, there is just one session, and, for others, it can be a weekly affair. The mechanics of a session are straightforward. There are three ways I administer ketamine: quick intravenous (IV) push, slow intravenous drip, and intramuscular injection. For first time patients, I use a 35 mg IV push. The slow IV drip is administered over 30 minutes and the dose varies from 50 to 80 mg. The intramuscular dose is given in the deltoid muscle in a dose of 50 to 60 mg. These have proven to be very safe dosages requiring no monitoring devices, and no patient has ever experienced any difficulties in terms of dosage. It is very important to discuss the ketamine experience in terms the patient can understand. I first explain this will be unlike any experience they have ever had, and it is very strong and unique. Going into it with comfort is essential. Being a first-time experience, it is natural to be anxious. "What will happen? Will I succeed or fail? Can I handle it?" This is an experience that cannot be controlled, and control freaks can have a real hard time letting go to the extent needed for the session. If, in speaking to such a one, they convey an inability or unwillingness to surrender control for the duration of the session (about 30 minutes), then I simply back away from using ketamine until they feel they can let the experience unfold.

I realized I needed to experience a "K" session myself, so I would know firsthand what it does and what one experiences. I quickly saw what this medicine does experientially. The details of its effects on neurotransmitters and on the brain interest me little, but I am happy others are looking into this aspect. I have always been interested in its practical applications, as this is the essence and focus of my clinical practice. In describing the experience of ketamine, we are all at a loss for words for reasons to which I will get. Often, the best we can do is to rely on metaphor; descriptions will vary depending on the person, their level of spiritual understanding, and their poetic inclination and ability. Within a minute of injecting the ketamine, a very odd sensation occurs. Many describe this as an OBE or out-of-body experience, and it is. It happens with such abruptness the patient needs to be prepared for this as best as possible. It is very important, at this moment, to recognize what is happening and to let go as much and as deeply as possible. It can feel like dying, and it is important prior to taking "K" that the patient understands they are *not* dying even though it may feel that way. All bodily functions continue to operate normally, and conscious awareness is not needed for the body to function during the session. While some experience their OBE as dying, others experience it as a great liberation, as if they have come home. These are the ones who don't want to come back. After the abrupt OBE, there follows an experience which varies between people and within the individual during multiple sessions. No two sessions are alike. Some are dark and others are very light. Within a session, some start out dark and then it all becomes very light. I have never seen it the other way around. Sometimes, there is a story, other times, a sequence of scenes, or geometric shapes, or bright colors. Sometimes, the feeling is blissful and expansive. Other times, it can be as if nothing happened. On questioning the latter type of non-experience, there will always be some nuggets to be extracted with a little digging and reflection.

Dark experiences are often followed by blissful ones, and the point must be made there is as much to gain from one as the other. I will allow some talk after a session, but only if the patient needs such. Once one does a session, this is an experience beyond the realm of words. It is unnecessary to talk afterward, and it sometimes serves to bring one out of their post "K" state of mind. One thing I have noticed is a complete absence of fear during the session, despite some anxiety going into it. It takes a week (sometimes even more), to integrate the experience. I always allow the patient to determine if more sessions are needed. It seems everyone knows if repeat sessions are needed, and they also know when their time with "K" is done. Careful explanation of what to expect must be accompanied by a safe, quiet, and serene setting. I prefer a more natural setting and find patients are very comfortable in such a setting. I dislike a clinical setting for a "K" session and all the monitoring devices and high-tech approaches I find unnecessary and only add to the expense.

What exactly is happening during a "K" session? Two key events take place. From a brain perspective, one experiences a "reset." This is a word coming from patients. This reset can allow a shift in the basic mood or affect; the default setting in the brain. If chronically depressed, one can see a change to less time being depressed or no depression at all. If it is PTSD the patient has, they can see the vanishing of that trauma, as if an eraser did its job on the part of the brain where the particular trauma memory was stored. This can happen in a single session, or some choose to do multiple sessions, each time getting the reset they so fervently desire and need.

The response is variable among individuals regarding duration of benefit. One gets an antidepressant effect and a reset with each session, and the effect seems to be cumulative. I know of no other modality that even approaches the profundity of ketamine's ability to reset the brain. While the brain reset is so beneficial and therapeutic, there is a parallel phenomenon that is more intriguing and profound. This is the OBE one experiences, and contextualizing this is important. One feels a complete loss of a sense of self. There is a temporary (15–30 minutes) loss of the mind/body, which we call the ego. A permanent loss of ego we know as death, and under the influence of ketamine, we get a sneak preview of what it will be like when we die. Most patients leave with a much more relaxed and less fearful attitude surrounding their death, perceiving there is a realm to which we return that seems to be eternal. This alone is worth the price of admission.

We are all entrapped within our ego and to be completely free of it for even a brief period is invariably liberating and instructive. Many have very amazing and fantastic journeys which can help inform their daily existence. If our ego disappears, what is it that is left? I recognize this as the realm of the soul, which we are oblivious to in our day-to-day existence. During the "K" experience, we get to visit the realm of pure soul unencumbered by ego. I know of no other means short of a near death experience that allows us this very special privilege. This visit to the realm of the soul will have many speak of coming home. Our true home to which we will permanently return upon the death of the body. This aspect of the journey also speaks to our true identity . . . "Who am I?" Most leave with a profound peace and sense of calm which often permeates their ego existence. In this age of anxiety, what could be better or more profound? When embarking on a ketamine journey, always send the prayer, "Connect with Source." You will.

Source: © Joel Friedman, MD.

Ketamine Foundations

Foundations such as the Ketamine Fund (www.ketaminefund.org) deserve special mention. Entrepreneurs and filmmakers Zappy Zapolin and Warren Gumpel founded the Ketamine Fund as a nonprofit organization that sponsors ketamine treatments for at-risk veterans. The goal of the Ketamine Fund is to bring down US veteran suicide rates by 70 percent. The Ketamine Fund has aligned with dozens of clinics to provide ketamine treatments to veterans. Their mission is to reach service members returning from duty experiencing severe mental trauma, such as suicidal thoughts. Zapolin vividly describes one veteran who was on twenty-two different medications from the VA hospital, and, after a series of ketamine treatments, he was able to stop all of his medications, go home, and have a relationship with his kids for the first time in ten years. These transitions happen fast, and you don't have to wait for weeks or months to see the effects. How else could one achieve this besides going to a country like Peru, sitting with a shaman, and experiencing deep integration with ayahuasca?

In an interview, Zapolin said his focus is on ketamine and how to make it more accessible to everyone. The current landscape shows ketamine is more accessible than other psychoactive agents, such as psilocybin and MDMA. Zapolin notes, "Psilocybin and MDMA have great potential, but they are not available throughout the country, whereas ketamine is available now. It's FDA approved, and hundreds of clinics use ketamine for depression and suicide." Warren Gumpel says ketamine saved his life as well. Before ketamine, he had considered suicide, and it was not until he found ketamine through Dr. Brooks in New York that he overcame his suicidal ideation.

Zapolin and Gumpel are the filmmakers behind the psychedelic advocacy film *The Reality of Truth* with actress Michelle Rodriguez and Dr. Deepak Chopra; it has been viewed millions of times since its release. Some have said things like, "I was going to commit suicide, then I saw this movie, and I started doing plant medicine, and it totally changed my life," and "I was a drug addict and homeless, and I found plant medicine through this movie." Zappy and Warren also recently produced *Lamar Odom: Reborn*, a movie about Lamar Odom's path to recovery. Odom played for the Los Angeles Lakers, winning championships in 2009 and 2010. He was also married to Khloe Kardashian for seven years. Battling mental illness and addiction, Lamar's life spiraled out of control in 2015 when he was found unconscious in a Nye County brothel in Nevada. On life support, Odom lived through multiple strokes and heart attacks while in the hospital and has been called a "walking miracle" by doctors. He survived a near lethal overdose and took action to seek treatment for patterns of addiction after years of trauma. The film highlights Lamar's journey using ketamine, plant medicines, and daily practice to overcome addiction, anxiety, and trauma.

Numerous telehealth startup companies emerged during the pandemic and played a critical role in expanding mental health access. Many provide at-home ketamine therapy with virtual guidance from licensed psychiatric doctors to achieve safe and successful outcomes with lower costs, more access, and greater convenience. The experience usually includes a video consultation to determine if ketamine therapy is appropriate. Then, a clinician discusses health history and goals for mental health treatment. If deemed a candidate, a kit is sent with oral ketamine, a blood pressure monitor, a meditation mask, and guidance on getting the most out of the experience. However, much controversy surrounds the telehealth medical model. Lawmakers fear telehealth companies will prescribe drugs with little oversight from management or qualified staff, possibly harming patients. Telehealth companies provide care to thousands of patients operating on the flexibilities implemented during the pandemic.

Better U, a national psychedelic therapy company, is a leading voice of mental health. Their goals are to end mental health stigmas and improve mental health access. Using a science-based approach, www.BetterUcare.com is one of many companies that prescribe at-home ketamine therapy, and many of their patients willingly share testimonials of their transformations. They are working towards reducing mental illness through broad forms of treatment, including psychiatry, psychotherapy, and psychedelic therapy. Their data (and many others) show improvements in over 80 percent of patients even after two sessions. The founders of BetterUcare.com, Derek Du Chesne and psychiatrist Dr. Sam Zand, highlight "raising awareness will decrease the discrimination and stigma against people with mental illness. This is why many people never seek help and end up taking their life." The Better U Foundation is working to provide subsidized, introductory ketamine therapy, emphasize lifestyle changes, and bridge access to psychiatric and psychedelic services. The foundation's spokesperson and cofounder is former professional baseball player and suicide survivor Drew Robinson, who was presented in an earlier chapter. Other co-founders include MLB manager of the year Gabe Kapler, NFL all-pro tight end

Darren Waller, UFC spokesperson Arianny Celeste, and Hollywood actress Catherine Oxenberg.

* * * *

Case Study: CEO of an IT Company (Anonymous)

Mr. A is a successful CEO of an international cybersecurity company. He is also a Vietnam veteran with significant PTSD. He explains that he has been using ketamine with his private physician for many years. The ketamine treatments helped him manage his PTSD and addiction, gain introspection, and open his mind, translating into better performance as a CEO and in his personal life. Mr. A recorded a detailed analysis of his ketamine experiences. He writes:

> The feeling of losing control is the beginning of the separation of mind, probably the neurons firing, a kind of "taking off." Last night, I discovered I still had the cognitive control to direct my mind in whatever I chased. I let go of my surroundings and thoughts influencing the direction and my cognitive thinking and chose to direct it deliberately to myself and my issues. I chose to focus the activity on my current stress and issues with all the things troubling me, and I could dissect my issues and rearrange them in another way. My happiness and health became the central core or the true intent that emerged as the director of the experience.
>
> I realized, after a bit, all these things troubling my life, so extreme, were my doing. To this point, I understood all I had to do was stop the way I had been embracing these problems and choose to let go of the unhealthy ways I dealt with them. Doing so would allow me to deal with these issues and be happy. At the same time, I was not delusional. I felt a new reality of these issues and how I have dealt with them in my reality, but without the stress. There are a bunch of things I need to handle, and I am capable of doing so. That creates my anxiety, fear, depression, and unhealthy responses. All I have to do is let go of these things within myself and keep

happiness and health as the center point. I can still perform and achieve and be healthy.

Furthermore, the result will be superior. This was a breakthrough in how I am supposed to manage the treatment experience and get the actual value out of it. This time was not a trippy experience that helped in other ways in the past. If the person doing the treatment understands what I learned last night, it can be of extraordinary benefit, well beyond what I have experienced before. I think I finally got it. What is unique about this treatment is it is not an uncontrolled trip. My mind still has control, and I can direct it. If a person doing this does not realize this or doesn't have any cognitive strength to do the treatment, it may not be good for them; that person will not be going into the treatment with a direct purpose and intent, and it will take you somewhere else.

For me, doing the treatment should start with a conducive and unobtrusive environment with a purpose on which you want to focus. Unlike other drugs you cannot control, this one you can. Even when the brain is firing off with force in a way you have never experienced, you still have fundamental control if you choose. You need to be aware of this; it is a bit tricky, but you have control. It is not acid!

* * * *

Ketamine Future and Beyond

Ketamine is the first antidepressant medication to be cleared by the FDA in many years. The excitement in the psychiatric community is clear, but one overbearing issue surrounding ketamine is cost and accessibility. The cost of ketamine infusions is out of reach for most people, and many must travel long distances. Insurance companies rarely reimburse ketamine treatments, except for Spravato, which must be preapproved and administered in an office setting. The recent interest in ketamine may bring psychedelic psychotherapy closer to the mainstream of psychiatry and neurology.

Other Psychedelics

Psychedelics like ayahuasca, MDMA, LSD, and psilocybin are gaining much attention in research studies and books. For example, Michael Pollan's *How to Change Your Mind* and *The Doors of Perception* by Aldous Huxley are popular books highlighting how drugs like LSD and psilocybin can give you a psychedelic experience and change your life. In *The Doors of Perception*, Huxley described his trial of mescaline as "the most extraordinary and significant experience available to human beings this side of the Beatific Vision."[4]

Psilocybin and other psychedelics have been used for centuries as sacraments within indigenous cultures. They were a focus within psychiatry as both probes of brain function and experimental therapeutics. By the late 1960s and early 1970s these scientific inquires fell out of favor because of governmental influence. However, sixty years later, scientific interest in classic psychedelics has returned and grown as a result of several promising studies, validating earlier research. Psilocybin, the drug in "magic" mushrooms, has been shown to be as effective as a common antidepressant, according to new research in *The New England Journal of Medicine*,[5] and a recent study from the Johns Hopkins School of Medicine on treating major depressive disorder with psilocybin-assisted therapy has shown excellent results.

Ketamine also provides this experience with a pharmaceutical-grade product in a controlled setting. Author and podcaster Tim Ferriss advocates psychedelic therapy with ketamine and psilocybin. Ferriss recently underwent a series of ketamine treatments for TRD. During his podcast with Dr. John Krystal, he was impressed by how it was possible not to have a loop or repetitive thought patterns. The subjective experience was tremendously therapeutic, especially during the treatment.

Dave Asprey, founder of Bulletproof Coffee, a company specializing in human optimization and bio-hacking, is no stranger to ketamine. Asprey has used ketamine and understands its positive effects on his brain. In a podcast about ketamine, Dave describes how one of his colleagues overcame her lifelong fear of needles with a single ketamine treatment. If she was presented with a needle, she fainted on the spot. While on ketamine, she could see the needle pushing on the IV catheter, and afterward, she said her fear was gone.

Conclusion

Ketamine is here to stay, but how we will move forward remains a question. We have seen many clinics, foundations, emergency departments, mental health hotlines, books, and more embrace the use of ketamine. Certainly, ketamine will move into the emergency departments and pediatric mental-health spaces. Pharmaceutical companies are developing derivatives of ketamine that avoid the psychoactive effects and preserve the mental health effects. Ketamine is moving out of the clinics and transitioning to home treatment through telehealth organizations. But most medical professionals strongly recommend it be administered by a physician.

Many physicians are open-minded to using ketamine for suicidal ideation; however, there are still some concerns. The primary issue is ketamine is a substantial drug of abuse worldwide. Despite the robust evidence showing that ketamine offers short- and long-term benefits to individuals suffering from suicidal ideations, this treatment has not yet undergone the multiple large-scale trials needed to determine the durability and safety of long-term treatment. Likely, they will never do these trials.

Yet, suicide is not going away. Given the worsening mental-health disparity, the continuing development of depression, and the increase in suicide ideation, it is vital to understand that alternatives exist and that we can save lives—possibly even your own. Psychedelics help us to detach from the normal patterns of life altogether. It helps us ask ourselves why we are doing this to ourselves, but without moral condemnation. Psychedelics help us understand things so that we do not have to repeat the actions continuously driving our minds.

As humans, we do not have any predators, and we only have ourselves to fear. Humans are unique in that we are the only species of animal that ever commits suicide, and about 2,000 do so every day. Researcher Darcia Narvaez writes humans are "species atypical," meaning that we uniquely create environments that hurt us. Humans are the only ones who will gratuitously and for no practical reason turn on each other, acting out of pure hatred and insanity. Honesty is the only way to approach our traumas because no future is possible without it. Ketamine is a game changer and is revolutionizing the treatment of mental illness. If you or a loved one are struggling with depression and suicidal ideation and have had little success with traditional treatments, ketamine may be the solution.

Useful Terms and Definitions

Before delving into how ketamine works, describing some of the terms involved is helpful.

Neuron: A brain cell. Neurons consist of a cell body (soma), dendrites, and axons. The cell body contains a nucleus and receives incoming electrical nerve impulses through dendrites and the axon, which are an extension of the neuron.

Synapse: A specialized structure that permits a neuron to pass an electrical or chemical signal to another neuron or other cell. The synapse is where all the action happens. Neurons release chemical neurotransmitters that diffuse across a small gap and activate special sites called receptors. Ketamine affects opioid, serotonin, cholinergic, and catecholamine receptors.

Neurotransmitters: The chemical messengers that transmit signals across a synapse from one neuron to another. Neurotransmitters are chemical substances made by the neuron specifically to transmit a message. Examples of neurotransmitters are glutamate, norepinephrine, epinephrine, serotonin, and many others.

Glutamate: The major excitatory neurotransmitter used by all living things and thought to be the most important in the brain. Over 80 percent of neurons have glutamate receptors, and they play important roles in cognitive functions, learning, and memory. One of the major actions of ketamine is to decrease or balance the action of glutamate.

GABA (Gamma-amino-butyric acid): The chief inhibitory neurotransmitter in the brain. Its principal role is to reduce neuronal excitability, and GABA is the opposite of glutamate.

NMDA receptor: NMDA stands for N-Methyl-D-aspartate. It is the glutamate receptor found in neurons, and it is activated when glutamate and glycine bind to it. This results in a positive flow of electrically charged signals through the cells. Many psychoactive drugs affect the NMDA receptor's activity, and ketamine blocks the NMDA receptors.

mTOR: The mechanistic target of rapamycin (mTOR). A protein made by cells that acts as a signaling pathway. Serves as a regulator of cell metabolism, growth, proliferation, and survival. Ketamine activates mTOR signaling in the brain.

BDNF: Brain Derived Neural Growth Factor (BDNF). Found in the brain and spinal cord, this protein promotes the survival of neurons by playing a role in the growth, maturation, and maintenance of brain cells. BDNF is responsible for plasticity in the brain, which is crucial for learning and memory. BDNF is increased by ketamine administration and certain types of exercise.

Epigenetic: This refers to heritable external modifications to a phenotype that do not change the DNA. Epigenetics is the reason a skin cell looks different from a brain cell. Epigenetic changes are said to come from the environment and may play a role in suicidality, meaning suicidal parents may pass genes to their children that may predispose them to suicide. An example could be the offspring of a person who produces less BDNF than normal people; thus, they may have a predisposition to depression and suicide.

Hippocampus: Named for its shape (from the Greek for "sea horse"), this structure is a major component of the brains of humans and other animals. The hippocampus is part of the limbic system and handles many bodily functions. The hippocampus is essential in storing long-term memories, response inhibition, and spatial cognition in the brain's center.

Prefrontal Cortex (PFC): This region of the brain covers the front part of the frontal lobe and is responsible for planning, personality expression, decision-making, and moderating social behavior. It is linked to a person's will to live, short-term memory, and specific aspects of speech and language. It is not fully mature until about twenty-five years of age in humans.

Electro-convulsive therapy (ECT): A medical procedure performed under anesthesia, where small electric currents are intentionally passed through the brain, triggering brief seizures. ECT is said to cause changes in brain chemistry, quickly reversing symptoms of certain medical health conditions. For an in-depth story about ECT, you can watch the TED Talk by Sherwin Nuland (https://www.ted.com/talks/sherwin_nuland_how_electroshock_therapy_changed_me).

Neuroplasticity: The brain can change through growth and reorganization, form new connections and pathways, and change how its circuits are wired. Once thought only to manifest during childhood, it is now known that adult brains demonstrate neuroplasticity. The adult brain is not entirely hard-wired, and new brain cells are formed even in adulthood.

Neurogenesis: The ability of the brain to grow new neurons or brain cells.

A Review of Ketamine Pharmacology

Ketamine belongs to the chemical class of drugs known as arylcyclohexylamines. In 1962, Professor Calvin Steven created a derivative of phencyclidine (PCP) called CI-581 through animal studies. The first human administration was in 1964, and they found it to produce dissociative anesthesia. The FDA approved ketamine for surgical anesthesia in 1970. Ketamine does not overly suppress breathing or blood pressure, which increased its popularity. It is often the only anesthetic in developing countries. In fact, the WHO labels it as an essential medicine because one can administer it without supplemental oxygen or a supply of electricity, which are necessary for the administration of many other anesthetics. Used as a "buddy drug" for injured soldiers, ketamine gained widespread use in the Vietnam War because a fellow soldier could administer it due to its relative safety. The US military still uses it today in the Middle East conflicts.

Ketamine is a mainstay for anesthesia and analgesia in veterinary medicine, and it is the only injectable anesthetic that is effective in a wide range of species. In the 1970s, ketamine hit the streets and was known by names like "Special K" and "Vitamin K." People who used ketamine and other psychedelics like LSD were known as "psychonauts." In the 1990s, ketamine abuse was evident, and efforts were made worldwide to limit illicit use. Lawmakers relabeled ketamine as a schedule 3 nonnarcotic substance under the US Controlled Substances Act. This further decreased studies of ketamine and psychiatric disorders. Ketamine's patent expired in 2002, so pharmaceutical companies had little incentive to study the drug.

Ketamine exists in two forms: the S (+) and the R (-) configurations. These are called enantiomers and exist as mirror images of each other. The S form is approximately twice as powerful as the R form. Distinguishing the different effects between the two forms is challenging. Current pharmacological preparations of ketamine comprise equal proportions of the two forms, a racemic mixture. The bioavailability of intramuscular (IM) ketamine is comparable to intravenous ketamine. A summary of the bioavailability is as follows: intravenous (100%), intramuscular (93%), nasal (25-50%), oral (17-24%), and sublingual (24-30%). The half-life of ketamine is one to three hours, meaning that half of the drug is eliminated from the body at this time. The subjective effects (euphoria, dissociation) cease quickly after the administration is stopped. The liver is metabolized into four distinct metabolites (hydroxynorketamine, dehydronorketamine, hydroxyketamine, and norketamine).

The specific stages of ketamine-altered states of consciousness exist as a function of drug dose. A low, sub-psychedelic dose (25 to 50 mg IM injection) resulted in an empathogenic experience characterized by happiness and increased body awareness. With a medium psychedelic dose (50 mg to 125 mg IM injection), people have out-of-body experiences, meaning that subjects feel completely separated from their bodies. Finally, in a high dose (150 to 200 mg IM injection), subjects undergo an ego-dissolving transcendental experience. In this state, individuals feel a dissolution of boundaries between the external reality and self and can have a "near-death" experience.

The Detailed Mechanism of How Ketamine Binds to Receptors

Ketamine binds to receptors in the cell lipid bilayer. These receptors are called "PCP" receptors for historical reasons. Just imagine these receptors are tunnels with a portion sticking into the cell and a portion sticking out of the cell. When ketamine binds to these receptors, it causes a blockage. The outer end of the tunnel is attached to a glutamate receptor, which is called an NMDA receptor, on the cell surface. The receptor complex is an NMDA –PCP or N-P receptor. The "N" part is on the outside and locks onto glutamate, and the "P" part is on the inside and locks onto ketamine. There are also binding sites for other chemicals, such as magnesium, to block the same tunnel. The complex is like a large space station with several docking bays for different spaceships.

It was once thought the P receptors were the same as PCP receptors, but now we know they are entirely distinct entities. The N-P receptor complex plays an important role in thinking, memory, emotion, language, sensation, and perception. Ketamine affects all of these areas, changing how incoming data is integrated.

A Technical Explanation of Ketamine and Neuroplasticity

Researchers believe ketamine increases brain synapses by increasing the proteins BDNF and mTOR. Both molecules rev up the synthesis of bio-molecules. Some of these biomolecules include lipids, proteins, and nucleotides. A more technical explanation of the mechanism of ketamine is in the interneurons in the prefrontal cortex, resulting in a surge of glutamate from the pyramidal neurons. Glutamate activates postsynaptic alpha-amino-3-hydroxy-5-methyl-4-isoxazole propionic acid receptors, which trigger the well-known mTOR-dependent protein synthesis and BDNF structural plasticity in the prefrontal cortex and hippocampus. A second hypothesis claims ketamine directly inhibits postsynaptic NMDA receptors on pyramidal neurons, which elicits the spontaneous release of glutamate, preventing the phosphorylation of eukaryotic elongation-factor-2 and resulting in rapid BDNF production. Animal studies show ketamine itself might target neuralplasticity independent of NMDA. These theories mentioned above converge on the activation of neuroplasticity via the activation of BDNF and mTOR pathways. BDNF is a major brain growth factor activating intracellular signaling cascades, one of them being mTOR, which regulates synaptic protein synthesis. The rapid increase of mTOR in the medial prefrontal cortex following ketamine administration results in local structural plasticity.

About the Author

Johnathan Edwards, MD, is a board-certified anesthesiologist with a key focus on treating mental-health conditions with ketamine. Dr. Edwards has provided ketamine in his practice for over twenty years. He works with psychiatrist Dr. Sam Zand to help patients with mental-health conditions.

Dr. Edwards is the author of several books and medical papers including *The Science of the Marathon*, *Chasing Dakar*—his study of the Dakar Rally—and *Suicide, COVID-19, and Ketamine*. He practices medicine in Las Vegas, Nevada, and Port Orange, Florida. Following his early career in motocross, he studied at Victor Valley Community College, the University of California at Davis, and Eastern Virginia Medical School. He later studied medicine in Lyon, France.

Dr. Edwards lives most of each year in Port Orange, Florida, with his wife and their daughter. A fluent French speaker, he and his family reside part-time in Provence.

For more information:
www.johnathanedwardsmd.com or www.docedwards.com

Sources

CHAPTER 2

Ezquerra-Romano, I. Ivan, W. Lawn, E. Krupitsky, and C. J. A. Morgan. "Ketamine for the Treatment of Addiction: Evidence and Potential Mechanisms." *Neuropharmacology* 142 (November 2018): 72–82. https://doi.org/10.1016/j.neuropharm.2018.01.017.

Grabski, Meryem, Amy McAndrew, Will Lawn, Beth Marsh, Laura Raymen, Tobias Stevens, Lorna Hardy, Fiona Warren, Michael Bloomfield, Anya Borissova, Emily Maschauer, Rupert Broomby, Robert Price, Rachel Coathup, David Gilhooly, Edward Palmer, Richard Gordon-Williams, Robert Hill, Jen Harris, O. Merve Mollaahmetoglu, Valerie Curran, Brigitta Brandner, Anne Lingford-Hughes, and Celia J. A. Morgan. "Adjunctive Ketamine with Relapse Prevention–Based Psychological Therapy in the Treatment of Alcohol Use Disorder." *American Journal of Psychiatry* 179, no. 2 (February 2022): 152–62. https://doi.org/10.1176/appi.ajp.2021.21030277.

Ko, Kwonmok, Gemma Knight, James J. Rucker, and Anthony J. Cleare. "Psychedelics, Mystical Experience, and Therapeutic Efficacy: A Systematic Review." *Frontiers in Psychiatry* 13 (July 2022): https://doi.org/10.3389/fpsyt.2022.917199.

Vargas, Maxemiliano V., Retsina Meyer, Arabo A. Avanes, Mark Rus, and David E. Olson. "Psychedelics and Other Psychoplastogens for Treating Mental Illness." *Frontiers in Psychiatry* 12 (October 2021): https://doi.org/10.3389/fpsyt.2021.727117.

Wilkinson, Samuel T., Elizabeth D. Ballard, Michael H. Bloch, Sanjay J. Mathew, James W. Murrough, Adriana Feder, Peter Sos, Gang Wang,

Carlos A. Zarate Jr., and Gerard Sanacora. "The Effect of a Single Dose of Intravenous Ketamine on Suicidal Ideation: A Systematic Review and Individual Participant Data Meta-Analysis." *American Journal of Psychiatry* 175, no. 2 (February 2018): 150–58. https://doi.org/10.1176/appi.ajp.2017.17040472.

CHAPTER 4

American Academy of Child and Adolescent Psychiatry. "Teen Suicide." Facts for Families, no. 10. Aacap.org, May 2008. https://www.aacap.org/AACAP/Families_and_Youth/Facts_for_Families/FFF-Guide/Teen-Suicide-10.aspx.

Anderson, Monica, and Jingjing Jiang. "Teens, Social Media and Technology 2018." Internet & Technology. Pew Research Center, May 31, 2018. https://www.pewresearch.org/internet/2018/05/31/teens-social-media-technology-2018/.

Centers for Disease Control and Prevention. *Morbidity and Mortality Weekly Report*, 64, no. 33 (August 28, 2015): https://stacks.cdc.gov/view/cdc/33051.

DeVille, Danielle C., Diana Whalen, Florence J. Breslin, Amanda S. Morris, Sahib S. Khalsa, Martin P. Paulus, and Deanna M. Barch. "Prevalence and Family-Related Factors Associated with Suicidal Ideation, Suicide Attempts, and Self-Injury in Children Aged 9 to 10 Years." *JAMA Network Open* 3, no. 2 (2020): https://doi.org/10.1001/jamanetworkopen.2019.20956.

Dwyer, Jennifer B., Chad Beyer, Samuel T. Wilkinson, Robert B. Ostroff, Zheala Qayyum, and Michael H. Bloch. "Ketamine as a Treatment for Adolescent Depression: A Case Report." *Journal of the American Academy of Child & Adolescent Psychiatry* 56, no. 4 (April 2017): 352–54. https://doi.org/10.1016/j.jaac.2017.01.006.

Guessoum, Sélim Benjamin, Jonathan Lachal, Rahmeth Radjack, Emilie Carretier, Sevan Minassian, Laelia Benoit, and Marie Rose Moro. "Adolescent Psychiatric Disorders during the COVID-19 Pandemic and Lockdown." *Psychiatry Research* 291 (September 2020): https://doi.org/10.1016/j.psychres.2020.113264.

Jones, Jason D., Rhonda C. Boyd, Monica E. Calkins, Annisa Ahmed, Tyler M. Moore, Ran Barzilay, Tami D. Benton, and Raquel E. Gur. "Parent-Adolescent Agreement about Adolescents' Suicidal Thoughts." *Pediatrics* 143, no. 2 (February 2019): https://doi.org/10.1542/peds.2018-1771.

Kailash Satyarthi Children's Foundation. *A Study on Impact of Lockdown and Economic Disruption on Poor Rural Households with Special Reference to Children.* New Delhi: Kailash Satyarthi Children's Foundation, 2020. https://satyarthi.org.in/wp-content/uploads/2020/LockDown%20Study%20Report.pdf.

Kim, Susan, Brittany S. Rush, and Timothy R. Rice. "A Systematic Review of Therapeutic Ketamine Use in Children and Adolescents with Treatment-Resistant Mood Disorders." *European Child & Adolescent Psychiatry* 30, no. 10 (2021): 1485–1501. https://doi.org/10.1007/s00787-020-01542-3.

Lee, Joyce. "Mental Health Effects of School Closures during COVID-19." *The Lancet Child & Adolescent Health* 4, no. 6 (June 2020): 421. https://doi.org/10.1016/S2352-4642(20)30109-7.

Li, Kuan, Guibao Zhou, Yan Xiao, Jiayu Gu, Qiuling Chen, Shouxia Xie, and Junyan Wu. "Risk of Suicidal Behaviors and Antidepressant Exposure among Children and Adolescents: A Meta-Analysis of Observational Studies." *Frontiers in Psychiatry* 13 (2022): https://doi.org/10.3389/fpsyt.2022.880496.

Lintern, Shaun. "Coronavirus Lockdown May Have Led to Increased Child Suicides, New Report Warns." *The Independent.* July 14, 2020. https://www.independent.co.uk/news/health/coronavirus-uk-child-suicide-mental-health-nhs-a9617671.html.

Lovelace, Berkeley, Jr., and Jasmine Kim. "CDC Warns Congress of 'Significant Public Health Consequences' if Schools Don't Reopen in the Fall." CNBC, July 31, 2020. https://www.cnbc.com/2020/07/31 /cdc-warns-congress-of-significant-public-health-consequences-if-schools -dont-reopen-in-the-fall.html.

Papolos, Demitri, Mark Frei, Daniel Rossignol, Steven Mattis, Laura C. Hernandez-Garcia, and Martin H. Teicher. "Clinical Experience Using Intranasal Ketamine in the Longitudinal Treatment of Juvenile Bipolar Disorder with Fear of Harm Phenotype." *Journal of Affective Disorders* 225 (January 2018): 545–51. https://doi.org/10.1016/j.jad.2017.08.081.

Pastor, Patricia, Cynthia Reuben, Catherine Duran, and LaJeana Hawkins. 2015. "Association between Diagnosed ADHD and Selected Characteristics among Children Aged 4-17 Years: United States, 2011-2013." *NCHS Data Brief*, no. 201 (May): 201. https://pubmed.ncbi.nlm.nih.gov/25974000/.

Ting, Sarah A., Ashley F. Sullivan, Edwin D. Boudreaux, Ivan Miller, and Carlos A. Camargo Jr. "Trends in US Emergency Department Visits for Attempted Suicide and Self-Inflicted Injury, 1993–2008." *General Hospital Psychiatry* 34, no. 5 (September-October 2012): 557–65. https://doi.org /10.1016/j.genhosppsych.2012.03.020.

Zarrinnegar, Paria, Jay Kothari, and Keith Cheng. "Successful Use of Ketamine for the Treatment of Psychotic Depression in a Teenager." *Journal of Child and Adolescent Psychopharmacology* 29, no. 6 (July 2019): 472–73. https://doi.org/10.1089/cap.2019.0028.

CHAPTER 5

Abdallah, Chadi G., John D. Roache, Ralitza Gueorguieva, Lynnette A. Averill, Stacey Young-McCaughan, Paulo R. Shiroma, Prerana Purohit, Antoinette Brundige, William Murff, Kyung-Heup Ahn, Mohamed A. Sherif, Eric J. Baltutis, Mohini Ranganathan, Deepak D'Souza, Brenda Martini, Steven M. Southwick, Ismene L. Petrakis, Rebecca R. Burson, Kevin B. Guthmiller, Argelio L. López-Roca, Karl A. Lautenschlager, John P. McCallin III, Matthew B. Hoch, Alexandar Timchenko, Sergio E. Souza, Charles E. Bryant, Jim Mintz, Brett T. Litz, Douglas E.

Williamson, Terence M. Keane, Alan L. Peterson, and John H. Krystal. "Dose-Related Effects of Ketamine for Antidepressant-Resistant Symptoms of Posttraumatic Stress Disorder in Veterans and Active Duty Military: A Double-Blind, Randomized, Placebo-Controlled Multi-Center Clinical Trial." *Neuropsychopharmacology* 47, no. 8 (July 2022): 1574–81. https://doi.org/10.1038/s41386-022-01266-9.

Lewiecki, E. Michael, and Sara A. Miller. "Suicide, Guns, and Public Policy." *American Journal of Public Health* 103, no. 1 (January 2013): 27–31. https://doi.org/10.2105/AJPH.2012.300964.

Ravindran, Chandru, Sybil W. Morley, Brady M. Stephens, Ian H. Stanley, and Mark A. Reger. "Association of Suicide Risk with Transition to Civilian Life among US Military Service Members." *JAMA Network Open* 3, no. 9 (2020): https://doi.org/10.1001/jamanetworkopen.2020.16261.

CHAPTER 6

Lu, Lin, Yuxia Fang, and Xi Wang. "Drug Abuse in China: Past, Present and Future." *Cellular and Molecular Neurobiology* 28, no. 4 (2008): 479–90. https://doi.org/10.1007/s10571-007-9225-2.

Rudd, Rose A., Noah Aleshire, Jon E. Zibbell, and R. Matthew Gladden. "Increases in Drug and Opioid Overdose Deaths—United States, 2000–2014." *Morbidity and Mortality Weekly Report* 64, no. 50 (January 1, 2016): 1378–82. https://doi.org/10.15585/mmwr.mm6450a3.

Schiller, Elizabeth Y., Amandeep Goyal, and Oren J. Mechanic. "Opioid Overdose." StatPearls (website), 2022. https://www.ncbi.nlm.nih.gov/books/NBK470415/.

CHAPTER 7

Allcott, Hunt, Luca Braghieri, Sarah Eichmeyer, and Matthew Gentzkow. "The Welfare Effects of Social Media." NEBR Working Paper Series 25514, National Bureau of Economic Research, Cambridge, MA, January 2019, revised November 2019. https://doi.org/10.3386/w25514.

Dy, Kiki. "Psychedelics and Sports: Can They Propel Athletes to Unprecedented Pinnacles of Ability?" Psychedelic Spotlight (website), October 20, 2021. https://psychedelicspotlight.com/psychedelics-sports -athletes-athletic-performance/.

Ostic, Dragana, Sikandar Ali Qalati, Belem Barbosa, Syed Mir Muhammad Shah, Esthela Galvan Vela, Ahmed Muhammad Herzallah, and Feng Liu. "Effects of Social Media Use on Psychological Well-Being: A Mediated Model." *Frontiers in Psychology* 12 (June 21, 2021): 678–766. https://doi .org/10.3389/fpsyg.2021.678766.

Watson, Clare. "The Psychedelic Remedy for Chronic Pain." *Nature* 609, no. 7929 (2022): 100–102. https://doi.org/10.1038/d41586-022-02878-3.

CHAPTER 8

Admon, Lindsay K., Vanessa K. Dalton, Giselle E. Kolenic, Susan L. Ettner, Anca Tilea, Rebecca L. Haffajee, Rebecca M. Brownlee, Melissa K. Zochowski, Karen M. Tabb, Maria Muzik, and Kara Zivin. "Trends in Suicidality 1 Year before and after Birth among Commercially Insured Childbearing Individuals in the United States, 2006–2017." *JAMA Psychiatry* 78, no. 2 (2021): 171–76. https://doi.org/10.1001/jamapsychiatry.2020.3550.

Admon, Roee, Mohammed R. Milad, and Talma Hendler. "A Causal Model of Post-Traumatic Stress Disorder: Disentangling Predisposed from Acquired Neural Abnormalities." *Trends in Cognitive Sciences* 17, no. 7 (July 2013): 337–47. https://doi.org/10.1016/j.tics.2013.05.005.

Anderson, George, and Michael Maes. "Schizophrenia: Linking Prenatal Infection to Cytokines, the Tryptophan Catabolite (TRYCAT) Pathway, NMDA Receptor Hypofunction, Neurodevelopment and Neuroprogression." *Progress in Neuro-Psychopharmacology and Biological Psychiatry* 42 (April 5, 2013): 5–19. https://doi.org/10.1016/j.pnpbp.2012.06.014.

Andrade, Chittaranjan. "Ketamine for Depression, 1: Clinical Summary of Issues Related to Efficacy, Adverse Effects, and Mechanism of Action."

Sources

Journal of Clinical Psychiatry 78, no. 4 (April 26, 2017): 415–19. https://doi
.org/10.4088/jcp.17f11567.

Bahr, Rebecca. "'Intranasal Esketamine (Spravato™) for Use in Treatment-
Resistant Depression in Conjunction with an Oral Antidepressant.'"
Pharmacy and Therapeutics 44, no. 6 (June 2019): 340–45. https://www
.ncbi.nlm.nih.gov/pmc/articles/PMC6534172/.

Ballard, Elizabeth D., David A. Luckenbaugh, Erica M. Richards, Tessa
L. Walls, Nancy E. Brutsché, Rezvan Ameli, Mark J. Niciu, Jennifer L.
Vande Voort, and Carlos A. Zarate Jr. "Assessing Measures of Suicidal
Ideation in Clinical Trials with a Rapid-Acting Antidepressant." *Journal of
Psychiatric Research* 68 (September 2015): 68–73. https://doi.org/10.1016/j
.jpsychires.2015.06.003.

Ballard, Elizabeth D., Dawn F. Ionescu, Jennifer L. Vande Voort, Mark
J. Niciu, Erica M. Richards, David A. Luckenbaugh, Nancy E. Brutsché,
Rezvan Ameli, Maura L. Furey, and Carlos A. Zarate. "Improvement in
Suicidal Ideation after Ketamine Infusion: Relationship to Reductions in
Depression and Anxiety." *Journal of Psychiatric Research* 58 (November
2014): 161–66. https://doi.org/10.1016/j.jpsychires.2014.07.027.

Haapanen, Laurell. "Ketamine Safe for Acutely Suicidal Patients in the
Emergency Department Setting." Psychiatry Advisor (website), December
5, 2019. https://www.psychiatryadvisor.com/home/depression-advisor/ketamine
-safe-for-acutely-suicidal-patients-in-the-emergency-department-setting/.

Haroon, Ebrahim, and Andrew H. Miller. "Inflammation Effects on Brain
Glutamate in Depression: Mechanistic Considerations and Treatment
Implications." *Current Topics in Behavioral Neurosciences* 31 (2017): 173–98.
https://doi.org/10.1007/7854_2016_40.

Irwin, Scott A., and Alana Iglewicz. "Oral Ketamine for the Rapid Treatment
of Depression and Anxiety in Patients Receiving Hospice Care." *Journal
of Palliative Medicine* 13, no. 7 (2010): 903–8. https://doi.org/10.1089/jpm
.2010.9808.

Janelidze, Shorena, Daniele Mattei, Åsa Westrin, Lil Träskman-Bendz, and Lena Brundin. "Cytokine Levels in the Blood May Distinguish Suicide Attempters from Depressed Patients." *Brain, Behavior, and Immunity* 25, no. 2 (February 2011): 335–39. https://doi.org/10.1016/j.bbi.2010.10.010.

Khan, Maryam S., Gwyneth W. Y. Wu, Victor I. Reus, Christina M. Hough, Daniel Lindqvist, Åsa Westrin, Brenton M. Nier, Owen M. Wolkowitz, and Synthia H. Mellon. "Low Serum Brain-Derived Neurotrophic Factor Is Associated with Suicidal Ideation in Major Depressive Disorder." *Psychiatry Research* 273 (March 2019): 108–13. https://doi.org/10.1016/j.psychres.2019.01.013.

Larkin, Gregory Luke, and Annette L. Beautrais. "A Preliminary Naturalistic Study of Low-Dose Ketamine for Depression and Suicide Ideation in the Emergency Department." *International Journal of Neuropsychopharmacology* 14, no. 8 (September 2011): 1127–31. https://doi.org/10.1017/s1461145711000629.

Li, Nanxin, Boyoung Lee, Rong-Jian Liu, Mounira Banasr, Jason M. Dwyer, Masaaki Iwata, Xiao-Yuan Li, George Aghajanian, and Ronald S. Duman. "MTOR-Dependent Synapse Formation Underlies the Rapid Antidepressant Effects of NMDA Antagonists." *Science* 329, no. 5994 (August 20, 2010): 959–64. https://doi.org/10.1126/science.1190287.

Li, Yanning, Ruipeng Shen, Gehua Wen, Runtao Ding, Ao Du, Jichuan Zhou, Zhibin Dong, Xinghua Ren, Hui Yao, Rui Zhao, Guohua Zhang, Yan Lu, and Xu Wu. "Effects of Ketamine on Levels of Inflammatory Cytokines IL-6, Il-1β, and TNF-α in the Hippocampus of Mice Following Acute or Chronic Administration." *Frontiers in Pharmacology* 8 (March 2017): 139. https://doi.org/10.3389/fphar.2017.00139.

Liebrenz, Michael, Rudolf Stohler, and Alain Borgeat. "Repeated Intravenous Ketamine Therapy in a Patient with Treatment-Resistant Major Depression." *World Journal of Biological Psychiatry* 10, no. 4-2 (2009): 640–43. https://doi.org/10.1080/15622970701420481.

Sources

Ma, Xian-cang, Peng Liu, Xiao-ling Zhang, Wen-hui Jiang, Min Jia, Cai-xia Wang, Ying-ying Dong, Yong-hui Dang, and Cheng-ge Gao. "Intranasal Delivery of Recombinant AAV Containing BDNF Fused with HA2TAT: A Potential Promising Therapy Strategy for Major Depressive Disorder." *Scientific Reports* 6, no. 1 (March 3, 2016): https://doi.org/10.1038/srep22404.

Price, Rebecca B., Matthew K. Nock, Dennis S. Charney, and Sanjay J. Mathew. "Effects of Intravenous Ketamine on Explicit and Implicit Measures of Suicidality in Treatment-Resistant Depression." *Biological Psychiatry* 66, no. 5 (September 1, 2009): 522–26. https://doi.org/10.1016/j.biopsych.2009.04.029.

Radvansky, Brian M., Khushbu Shah, Anant Parikh, Anthony N. Sifonios, Vanny Le, and Jean D. Eloy. "Role of Ketamine in Acute Postoperative Pain Management: A Narrative Review." *BioMed Research International* 2015 (2015): 1–10. https://doi.org/10.1155/2015/749837.

Zarate, Carlos A., Jr., Jaskaran B. Singh, Paul J. Carlson, Nancy E. Brutsche, Rezvan Ameli, David A. Luckenbaugh, Dennis S. Charney, and Husseini K. Manji. "A Randomized Trial of an N-Methyl-D-Aspartate Antagonist in Treatment-Resistant Major Depression." *Archives of General Psychiatry* 63, no. 8 (2006): 856–64. https://doi.org/10.1001/archpsyc.63.8.856.

CHAPTER 9

"Correction to 'Psychedelics.'" *Pharmacological Reviews* 68, no. 2 (April 2016): 356. https://doi.org/10.1124/pr.114.011478err.

McIntyre, Roger S., Joshua D. Rosenblat, Charles B. Nemeroff, Gerard Sanacora, James W. Murrough, Michael Berk, Elisa Brietzke, Seetal Dodd, Philip Gorwood, Roger Ho, Dan V. Iosifescu, Carlos Lopez Jaramillo, Siegfried Kasper, Kevin Kratiuk, Jung Goo Lee, Yena Lee, Leanna M. W. Lui, Rodrigo B. Mansur, George I. Papakostas, Mehala Subramaniapillai, Michael Thase, Eduard Vieta, Allan H. Young, Carlos Zarate Jr., and Stephen Stahl. "Synthesizing the Evidence for Ketamine and Esketamine in Treatment-Resistant Depression: An International Expert Opinion on the Available Evidence and Implementation." *American Journal of Psychiatry* 178, no. 5 (May 1, 2021): 383–99. https://doi.org/10.1176/appi .ajp.2020.20081251.

Murrough, J. W., L. Soleimani, K. E. DeWilde, K. A. Collins, K. A. Lapidus, B. M. Iacoviello, M. Lener, M. Kautz, J. Kim, J. B. Stern, R. B. Price, A. M. Perez, J. W. Brallier, G. J. Rodriguez, W. K. Goodman, D. V. Iosifescu, and D. S. Charney. "Ketamine for Rapid Reduction of Suicidal Ideation: A Randomized Controlled Trial." *Psychological Medicine* 45, no. 16 (December 2015): 3571–80. https://doi.org/10.1017/s0033291715001506.

Endnotes

FOREWORD
1. Krystal, John H., Chadi G. Abdallah, Gerard Sanacora, Dennis S. Charney, and Ronald S. Duman. "Ketamine: A Paradigm Shift for Depression Research and Treatment." *Neuron* 101, no. 5 (March 6, 2019): 774–78. https://doi.org/10.1016/j .neuron.2019.02.005.

CHAPTER 1
1. Insel, Thomas, in discussion with the author, July 2021.
2. World Health Organization. "Suicide in the US (2019 Data)." American Association of Suicidology, last updated January 2021. https://suicidology.org/facts-and-statistics/.
3. Dastagir, Alia E. "More and More Americans Are Dying by Suicide. What Are We Missing?" *USA Today*, January 30, 2020. https://www.usatoday.com/story/news/nation /2020/01/30/u-s-suicide-rate-rose-again-2018-how-can-suicide-prevention-save -lives/4616479002/.
4. Garnett, Matthew F., Sally C. Curtin, and Deborah M. Stone. "Suicide Mortality in the United States, 2000–2020." *NCHS Data Brief*, no. 433 (March 2022): 1–8. https://dx.doi.org/10.15620/cdc:114217.
5. Stone, Deborah M., Thomas R. Simon, Katherine A. Fowler, Scott R. Kegler, Keming Yuan, Kristin M. Holland, Asha Z. Ivey-Stephenson, and Alex E. Crosby. "Vital Signs: Trends in State Suicide Rates—United States, 1999–2016 and Circumstances Contributing to Suicide—27 States, 2015." *Morbidity and Mortality Weekly Report* 67, no. 22 (June 8, 2018): 617–24. https://doi.org/10.15585/mmwr.mm6722a1.
6. Preti, Antonio. "Suicide among Animals: A Review of Evidence." Pt. 1. *Psychological Reports* 101, no. 3 (2007): 831–48. https://doi.org/10.2466/pr0.101.3.831-848.
7. Chalabi, Mona. "How Bad Is US Gun Violence? These Charts Show the Scale of the Problem." *The Guardian*. October 5, 2017. http://www.theguardian.com/us-news /2017/oct/05/us-gun-violence-charts-data.
8. World Health Organization. "Suicide in the US (2019 Data)."
9. Dastagir. "More Americans Are Dying by Suicide."
10. Dastagir.
11. Garnett, Curtin, and Stone. "Suicide Mortality in the United States."
12. Chalabi. "How Bad Is US Gun Violence?"

13. Schippers, Michaéla C. "For the Greater Good? The Devastating Ripple Effects of the Covid-19 Crisis." *Frontiers in Psychology* 11 (September 2020): https://doi.org/10.3389/fpsyg.2020.577740.
14. Schippers.
15. Chalabi. "How Bad Is US Gun Violence?"
16. Schippers. "For the Greater Good?"
17. Ahmad, Farida B., and Robert N. Anderson. "The Leading Causes of Death in the US for 2020." *Journal of the American Medical Association* 325, no. 18 (2021): 1829–30. https://doi.org/10.1001/jama.2021.5469.
18. Sidhu, Sabrina. "UNICEF: An Additional 6.7 Million Children under 5 Could Suffer from Wasting This Year Due to COVID-19." Unicef.org, July 27, 2020. https://www.unicef.org/press-releases/unicef-additional-67-million-children-under-5-could-suffer-wasting-year-due-covid-19.
19. World Health Organization. *World Malaria Report 2021.* Geneva: World Health Organization, December 2021. https://www.who.int/teams/global-malaria-programme/reports/world-malaria-report-2021.
20. Tjaden, Patricia, and Nancy Thoennes. *Full Report of the Prevalence, Incidence, and Consequences of Violence against Women.* Washington, DC: US Department of Justice, November 2000. https://www.ojp.gov/pdffiles1/nij/183781.pdf.
21. Brådvik, Louise. "Suicide Risk and Mental Disorders." *International Journal of Environmental Research and Public Health* 15, no. 9 (September 2018): 2028. https://doi.org/10.3390/ijerph15092028.
22. Stix, Gary. "From Club to Clinic: Physicians Push Off-Label Ketamine as Rapid Depression Treatment." Pt. 1. *Talking Back* (blog). *Scientific American*, September 11, 2013. https://blogs.scientificamerican.com/talking-back/from-club-to-clinic-physicians-push-off-label-ketamine-as-rapid-depression-treatment-part-1/.
23. Kritzer, Michael D., Nicholas A. Mischel, Jonathan R. Young, Christopher S. Lai, Prakash S. Masand, Steven T. Szabo, and Sanjay J. Mathew. "Ketamine for Treatment of Mood Disorders and Suicidality: A Narrative Review of Recent Progress." *Annals of Clinical Psychiatry* 34, no. 1 (February 2022): 33–43. https://doi.org/10.12788/acp.0048.
24. Duman, Ronald S., and George K. Aghajanian. "Synaptic Dysfunction in Depression: Potential Therapeutic Targets." *Science* 338, no. 6103 (October 5, 2012): 68–72. https://doi.org/10.1126/science.1222939.
25. Velasquez-Manoff, Moises. "Ketamine Stirs Up Hope—and Controversy—as a Depression Drug." *Wired*, May 8, 2018. https://www.wired.com/story/ketamine-stirs-up-hope-controversy-as-a-depression-drug/.
26. Wolfson, Phil, and Glenn Hartelius. *The Ketamine Papers: Science, Therapy, and Transformation.* Santa Cruz, CA: Multidisciplinary Association for Psychedelic Studies, 2016.
27. Oxenberg, Catherine. *Captive: A Mother's Crusade to Save Her Daughter from a Terrifying Cult.* New York: Gallery Books, 2018.
28. Brådvik. "Suicide Risk and Mental Disorders."

Endnotes

29. Maté, Gabor, and Daniel Maté. *The Myth of Normal: Trauma, Illness, & Healing in a Toxic Culture*. New York: Penguin Audio, 2022. Audio ed., 18 hr., 13 min.
30. Becker, Gavin de. *The Gift of Fear: Survival Signals That Protect Us from Violence*. London: Bloomsbury Publishing, 2000.
31. Velasquez-Manoff. "Ketamine Stirs Up Hope."
32. Du Chesne, Derek, in discussion with the author, 2023.

CHAPTER 2

1. Li, Linda, and Phillip E. Vlisides. "Ketamine: 50 Years of Modulating the Mind." *Frontiers in Human Neuroscience* 10 (November 2016): 1–15. https://doi.org/10.3389/fnhum.2016.00612.
2. Dai, Danika, Courtney Miller, Violeta Valdivia, Brian Boyle, Paula Bolton, Shuang Li, Steve Seiner, and Robert Meisner. "Neurocognitive Effects of Repeated Ketamine Infusion Treatments in Patients with Treatment Resistant Depression: A Retrospective Chart Review." *BMC Psychiatry* 22, no. 1 (2022): https://doi.org/10.1186/s12888-022-03789-3.
3. Krystal, John H., Chadi G. Abdallah, Gerard Sanacora, Dennis S. Charney, and Ronald S. Duman. "Ketamine: A Paradigm Shift for Depression Research and Treatment." *Neuron* 101, no. 5 (2019): 774–78. https://doi.org/10.1016/j.neuron.2019.02.005.
4. Yensen, Richard. "Psychedelic Experiential Pharmacology: Pioneering Clinical Explorations with Salvador Roquet (How I Came to All of This: Ketamine, Admixtures and Adjuvants, Don Juan and Carlos Castaneda Too): An Interview with Richard Yensen." Interview by Philip E. Wolfson. *International Journal of Transpersonal Studies* 33, no. 2 (July 2014): 160–74. https://doi.org/10.24972/ijts.2014.33.2.160.
5. *The Times*. World in Brief, January 30, 2004. www.thetimes.co.uk.
6. Mills, I. H., G. R. Park, A. R. Manara, and R. J. Merriman. "Treatment of Compulsive Behaviour in Eating Disorders with Intermittent Ketamine Infusions." *QJM: An International Journal of Medicine* 91, no. 7 (July 1998): 493–503. https://doi.org/10.1093/qjmed/91.7.493.
7. Berman, Robert M., Angela Cappiello, Amit Anand, Dan A. Oren, George R. Heninger, Dennis S. Charney, and John H. Krystal. "Antidepressant Effects of Ketamine in Depressed Patients." *Biological Psychiatry* 47, no. 4 (2000): 351–54. https://doi.org/10.1016/s0006-3223(99)00230-9.
8. Berman et al.
9. Yansen, "Psychedelic Experiential Pharmacology."
10. Domino, Edward F., David S. Warner. "Taming the Ketamine Tiger." *Anesthesiology* 113 (September 2010): 678–84. https://doi.org/10.1097/ALN.0b013e3181ed09a2.
11. National Institute of Mental Health. "Major Depression." Last modified January 2022. https://www.nimh.nih.gov/health/statistics/major-depression.
12. Berman et al. "Antidepressant Effects of Ketamine."
13. Zarate, Carlos A., Jr, Jaskaran B. Singh, Paul J. Carlson, Nancy E. Brutsche, Rezvan Ameli, David A. Luckenbaugh, Dennis S. Charney, and Husseini K. Manji. "A Randomized Trial of an N-Methyl-D-Aspartate Antagonist in Treatment-Resistant

Major Depression." *Archives of General Psychiatry* 63, no. 8 (2006): 856–64. https://doi.org/10.1001/archpsyc.63.8.856.

14. Dai et al. "Neurocognitive Effects of Repeated Ketamine Infusion."

15. Can, Adem T., Daniel F. Hermens, Megan Dutton, Cyrana Gallay, Emma Jensen, Monique Jones, Jennifer Scherman, Denise A. Beaudequin, Cian Yang, Paul E. Schwenn, and Jim Lagopoulos. "Low Dose Oral Ketamine Treatment in Chronic Suicidality: An Open-Label Pilot Study." *Translational Psychiatry* 11 (February 2021): https://doi.org/10.1038/s41398-021-01230-z.

16. Bolwig, Tom G., and Max Fink. "Electrotherapy for Melancholia: The Pioneering Contributions of Benjamin Franklin and Giovanni Aldini." *Journal of Electroconvulsive Therapy* 25, no. 1 (March 2009): 15–18. https://pubmed.ncbi.nlm.nih.gov/19209070/.

17. Li and Vlisides. "Ketamine: 50 Years of Modulating the Mind."

18. Zarate et al. "A Randomized Trial of an N-Methyl-D-Aspartate."

19. Price, Rebecca B., Matthew K. Nock, Dennis S. Charney, Sanjay Mathew. "Effects of Intravenous Ketamine on Explicit and Implicit Measures of Suicidality in Treatment-Resistant Depression." *Biological Psychiatry* 66, no. 5 (September 2009): 522–26. https://doi.org/10.1016/j.biopsych.2009.04.029.

20. Liebrenz, Michael, Rudolf Stohler, and Alain Borgeat. "Repeated Intravenous Ketamine Therapy in a Patient with Treatment-Resistant Major Depression." *World Journal of Biological Psychiatry* 10, no. 4-2 (2009): 640–43. https://doi.org/10.1080/15622970701420481.

21. Bhojani, Fatima. "A Recovery Story: After Every Available Option Was Exhausted, Ketamine Has Enabled Her Life to Resume." Brain & Behavior Research Foundation (website), March 31, 2019. https://www.bbrfoundation.org/blog/recovery-story-after-every-available-option-was-exhausted-ketamine-has-enabled-her-life-resume.

22. Calabrese, Lori. "Titrated Serial Ketamine Infusions Stop Outpatient Suicidality and Avert ER Visits and Hospitalizations." *International Journal of Psychiatry Research* 2, no. 6 (2019): 1–12. https://doi.org/10.33425/2641-4317.1033.

23. Domany, Yoav, Richard C. Shelton, and Cheryl B. McCullumsmith. "Ketamine for Acute Suicidal Ideation. An Emergency Department Intervention: A Randomized, Double-Blind, Placebo-Controlled, Proof-of-Concept Trial." *Depression and Anxiety* 37, no. 3 (March 2020): 224–33. https://doi.org/10.1002/da.22975.

24. Ketamine Research Institute. "Olive's View of Heaven," February 13, 2019. https://ketamineinstitute.com/depression/olives-view-of-heaven/.

25. Krupitsky, E. M., and A. Y. Grinenko. "Ketamine Psychedelic Therapy (KPT): A Review of the Results of Ten Years of Research." *Journal of Psychoactive Drugs* 29, no. 2 (1997): 165–83. https://doi.org/10.1080/02791072.1997.10400185.

26. Ezquerra-Romano, I. Ivan, W. Lawn, E. Krupitsky, and C. J. A. Morgan. "Ketamine for the Treatment of Addiction: Evidence and Potential Mechanisms." *Neuropharmacology* 142 (November 2018): 72–82. https://doi.org/10.1016/j.neuropharm.2018.01.017.

27. Feder, Adriana, Sara Costi, Sarah B. Rutter, Abigail B. Collins, Usha Govindarajulu, Manish K. Jha, Sarah R. Horn, Marin Kautz, Morgan Corniquel, Katherine A. Collins, Laura Bevilacqua, Andrew M. Glasgow, Jess Brallier, Robert H. Pietrzak, James W. Murrough, and Dennis S. Charney. "A Randomized Controlled Trial of

Endnotes

Repeated Ketamine Administration for Chronic Posttraumatic Stress Disorder." *American Journal of Psychiatry* 178, no. 2 (February 2021): 193–202. https://doi.org /10.1176/appi.ajp.2020.20050596.

28. Donoghue, Anna C., Mark G. Roback, and Kathryn R. Cullen. "Remission from Behavioral Dysregulation in a Child with PTSD after Receiving Procedural Ketamine." *Pediatrics* 136, no. 3 (2015): e694-96. https://doi.org/10.1542/peds.2014-4152.

29. Mitchell, Jennifer M., Michael Bogenschutz, Alia Lilienstein, Charlotte Harrison, Sarah Kleiman, Kelly Parker-Guilbert, Marcela Ot'alora, Wael Garas, Casey Paleos, Ingmar Gorman, Christopher Nicholas, Michael Mithoefer, Shannon Carlin, Bruce Poulter, Ann Mithoefer, Sylvestre Quevedo, Gregory Wells, Sukhpreet S. Klaire, Bessel van der Kolk, Keren Tzarfaty, Revital Amiaz, Ray Worthy, Scott Shannon, Joshua D. Woolley, Cole Marta Yevgeniy Gelfand, Emma Hapke, Simon Amar, Yair Wallach, Randall Brown, Scott Hamilton, Julie B. Wang, Allison Coker, Rebecca Matthews, Alberdina de Boer, Berra Yazar-Klosinski, Amy Emerson, and Rick Doblin. "MDMA-Assisted Therapy for Severe PTSD: A Randomized, Double-Blind, Placebo-Controlled Phase 3 Study." *Nature Medicine* 27 (2021): 1025–33. https://doi .org/10.1038/s41591-021-01336-3.

30. Ross, Cassie, Rakesh Jain, Carl J. Bonnett, and Philip Wolfson. "High-Dose Ketamine Infusion for the Treatment of Posttraumatic Stress Disorder in Combat Veterans." *Annals of Clinical Psychiatry* 31, no. 4 (November 2019): 271–79. https://pubmed.ncbi .nlm.nih.gov/31675388/.

31. Clark, J. David. "Ketamine for Chronic Pain: Old Drug New Trick?" *Anesthesiology* 133, no. 1 (July 2020): 13–15. https://doi.org/10.1097/aln.0000000000003342.

32. Radvansky Brian M., Khusbu Shah, Anant Parikh, Anthoiny N. Sifonios, Vanny Le, and Jean D. Eloy. "Role of Ketamine in Acute Postoperative Pain Management: A Narrative Review." *BioMed Research International 2015* (2015): https://doi.org /10.1155/2015/749837.

33. Clark. "Ketamine for Chronic Pain."

34. Ferriss, Tim. "Dr. John Krystal—All Things Ketamine, the Most Comprehensive Podcast Episode Ever." *The Tim Ferriss Show*. Sept 30, 2022. Podcast, 3 hr., 54 min. https: //podcasts.apple.com/us/podcast/625-dr-john-krystal-all-things-ketamine-the-most /id863897795?i=1000581086124.

35. Ignaszewski, Martha J., Kaizad Munshi, Jason Fogler, and Marilyn Augustyn. "Transitions, Suicidality, and Underappreciated Autism Spectrum Disorder in a High School Student." *Journal of Developmental & Behavioral Pediatrics* 40, no 7 (September 2019): 563–65. https://doi.org/10.1097/DBP.0000000000000717.

36. Cassidy, Sarah, and Jacqui Rodgers. "Understanding and Prevention of Suicide in Autism." *Lancet Psychiatry* 4, no. 6 (June 2017): https://doi.org/10.1016/S2215 -0366(17)30162-1.

37. Danforth, Alicia L., Charles S. Grob, Christopher Struble, Allison A. Feducia, Nick Walker, Lisa Jerome, Berra Yazar-Klosinski, and Amy Emerson. "Reduction in Social Anxiety after MDMA-Assisted Psychotherapy with Autistic Adults: A Randomized, Double-Blind, Placebo-Controlled Pilot Study." *Psychopharmacology* 235 (2018): 3137–48. https://doi.org/10.1007/s00213-018-5010-9.

38. Hughes, Rebecca B., Jayde Whittingham-Dowd, Rachel E. Simmons, Steven J. Clapcote, Susan J. Broughton, and Neil Dawson. "Ketamine Restores Thalamic-Prefrontal Cortex Functional Connectivity in a Mouse Model of Neurodevelopmental Disorder-Associated 2p16.3 Deletion." *Cerebral Cortex Communications* 30, no. 4 (April 2020):2358–71. https://doi.org/10.1093/cercor/bhz244.

39. Kolevzon, Alexander, Tess Levy, Sarah Barkley, Sandra Bedrosian-Sermone, Matthew Davis, Jennifer Foss-Feig, Danielle Halpern, Katherine Keller, Ana Kostic, Christina Layton, Rebecca Lee, Bonnie Lerman, Matthew Might, Sven Sandin, Paige M. Siper, Laura G. Sloofman, Hannah Walker, Jessica Zweifach, and Joseph D. Buxbaum. "An Open-Label Study Evaluating the Safety, Behavioral, and Electrophysiological Outcomes of Low-Dose Ketamine in Children with ADNP Syndrome." *Human Genetics and Genomics Advances* 3, no. 4 (October 2022): https://doi.org/10.1016/j .xhgg.2022.100138.

40. Wink, Logan K., Debra L. Reisinger, Paul Horn, Rebecca C. Shaffer, Kaela O'Brien, Lauren Schmitt, Kelli R. Dominick, Ernest V. Pedapati, and Craig A. Erickson. "Brief Report: Intranasal Ketamine in Adolescents and Young Adults with Autism Spectrum Disorder—Initial Results of a Randomized, Controlled, Crossover, Pilot Study." *Journal of Autism and Developmental Disorders* 51, no. 4 (April 2021): 1392–99. https://doi.org/10.1007/s10803-020-04542-z.

41. Danforth, Alicia. "Psychedelic-Assisted Therapy for Social Adaptability in Autistic Adults." In *Disruptive Psychopharmacology*, eds. F. S. Barrett and K. H. Preller, 71–92. Vol. 56 of *Current Topics in Behavioral Neurosciences*. Cham, Switzerland: Springer, 2022. https://doi.org/10.1007/7854_2021_269.

42. Orsini, Aaron, in discussion with the author, February 2023. See https://www .AutisticPsychedelic.com.

43. Vargas, Maximiliano V., Retsina Meyer, Arabo A. Avanes, Mark Rus, and David E. Olson. "Psychedelics and Other Psychoplastogens for Treating Mental Illness." *Frontiers in Psychiatry* 12 (October 2021): https://doi.org/10.3389/fpsyt.2021.727117.

44. Maltbie, Eric A., Gopinath S. Kaundinya, and Leonard L. Howell. "Ketamine and Pharmacological Imaging: Use of Functional Magnetic Resonance Imaging to Evaluate Mechanisms of Action." *Behavioural Pharmacology* 28, no. 8 (2017): 610–22. https://doi.org/10.1097/fbp.0000000000000354.

45. Hase Arian, Max Erdmann, Verena Limbach, and Gregor Hasler. "Analysis of Recreational Psychedelic Substance Use Experiences Classified by Substance." *Psychopharmacology* 239, no. 2 (February 2022): 643–59. https://doi.org/10.1007 /s00213-022-06062-3.

46. Davis, Alan K., Frederick S. Barrett, Darrick G. May, Mary P. Cosimano, Nathan D. Sepeda, Matthew W. Johnson, Patrick H. Finan, and Roland R. Griffiths. "Effects of Psilocybin-Assisted Therapy on Major Depressive Disorder: A Randomized Clinical Trial." *JAMA Psychiatry* 78, no. 5 (2021): 481–89. https://doi.org/10.1001 /jamapsychiatry.2020.3285.

47. Krupitsky, E. M., and A. Y. Grinenko. "Ketamine Psychedelic Therapy (KPT): A Review of the Results of Ten Years of Research." *Journal of Psychoactive Drugs* 29, no. 2 (1997): 165–83. https://doi.org/10.1080/02791072.1997.10400185.

48. Orhurhu, Vwaire J., Rishik Vashisht, Lauren E. Claus, and Steven P. Cohen. "Ketamine Toxicity." StatPearls (website), 2022. https://www.ncbi.nlm.nih.gov/books /NBK541087/.

CHAPTER 3

1. Van Orden, Kimberly A., Tracy K. Witte, Kelly C. Cukrowicz, Scott R. Braithwaite, Edward A. Selby, and Thomas E. Joiner Jr. "The Interpersonal Theory of Suicide." *Psychological Review* 117, no. 2 (2010): 575–600. https://doi.org/10.1037/a0018697.

2. Ting, Sarah A., Ashley F. Sullivan, Edwin D. Boudreaux, Ivan Miller, and Carlos A. Camargo Jr. "Trends in US Emergency Department Visits for Attempted Suicide and Self-Inflicted Injury, 1993–2008." *General Hospital Psychiatry* 34, no. 5 (September-October 2012): 557–65. https://doi.org/10.1016/j.genhosppsych.2012.03.020.

3. US Public Health Service. *National Strategy for Suicide Prevention: Goals and Objectives for Action.* Washington, DC: Department of Health and Human Services, 2001.

4. US Public Health Service.

5. Barr, Ben, David Taylor-Robinson, Alex Scott-Samuel, Martin McKee, and David Stuckler. "Suicides Associated with the 2008–10 Economic Recession in England: Time Trend Analysis." *BMJ* 345, (2012): https://doi.org/10.1136/bmj.e5142.

6. Harper, Sam, Thomas J. Charters, Erin C. Strumpf, Sandro Galea, and Arijit Nandi. "Economic Downturns and Suicide Mortality in the USA, 1980–2010: Observational Study." *International Journal of Epidemiology* 44, no. 3 (June 2015): 956–66. https: //doi.org/10.1093/ije/dyv009.

7. Sakamoto, Haruka, Masahiro Ishikane, Cyrus Ghaznavi, and Peter Ueda. "Assessment of Suicide in Japan during the COVID-19 Pandemic vs. Previous Years." *JAMA Network Open* 4, no. 2 (February 2021): https://doi.org/10.1001 /jamanetworkopen.2020.37378.

8. Sakamoto, Ishikane, Ghaznavi, and Ueda.

9. Ohto, Hitoshi, Masaharu Maeda, Hirooki Yabe, Seiji Yasumura, and Evelyn E. Bromet. "Suicide Rates in the Aftermath of the 2011 Earthquake in Japan." *The Lancet* 385, no. 9979 (May 2, 2015): 1727. https://doi.org/10.1016/S0140-6736(15)60890-X.

10. Wilson, Greg. "Exec Of Major Retailer Dies in Plunge from NYC Hi-Rise as Firm Plans Mass Firings." Daily Wire (website), September 4, 2022. https://www.dailywire .com/news/exec-of-major-retailer-dies-in-plunge-from-nyc-hi-rise-as-firm-plans -mass-firings.

11. Benen, Steve. "For 19th Straight Week, Unemployment Filings Top 1 Million." *MaddowBlog.* MSNBC, July 30, 2020. https://www.msnbc.com/rachel-maddow-show /maddowblog/19th-straight-week-unemployment-filings-top-1-million-n1235299.

12. Berrenson, Alex. *Unreported Truths About COVID-19 and Lockdowns.* Vol. 1. Self-published, Bowker, June 4, 2020.

13. Iob, Eleonora, Andrew Steptoe, and Daisy Fancourt. "Abuse, Self-Harm and Suicidal Ideation in the UK during the COVID-19 Pandemic." *British Journal of Psychiatry* 217, no. 4 (2020): 543–46. https://doi.org/10.1192/bjp.2020.130.

14. Travis-Lumer, Yael, Arad Kodesh, Yair Goldberg, Sophia Frangou, and Stephen Z. Levine. "Attempted Suicide Rates before and during the COVID-19 Pandemic:

Interrupted Time Series Analysis of a Nationally Representative Sample." *Psychological Medicine* (2021): 1–7. https://doi.org/10.1017/S0033291721004384.

15. Travis-Lumer et al.
16. Reger, Mark A., Ian H. Stanley, and Thomas E. Joiner. "Suicide Mortality and Coronavirus Disease 2019—A Perfect Storm?" *JAMA Psychiatry* 77, no. 11 (2020): 1093–94. https://doi.org/10.1001/jamapsychiatry.2020.1060.
17. Ohto et al. "Suicide Rates in Aftermath of 2011 Earthquake."
18. American Association of Suicidology. "American Association of Suicidology Addresses Suicide Rate During Novel Coronavirus Pandemic," news release, November 2, 2020. https://suicidology.org/2020/11/02/covidandsuicide/.
19. Jones, Jason D., Rhonda C. Boyd, Monica E. Calkins, Annisa Ahmed, Tyler M. Moore, Ran Barzilay, Tami D. Benton, and Raquel E. Gur. "Parent-Adolescent Agreement about Adolescents' Suicidal Thoughts." *Pediatrics* 143, no. 2 (February 2019): https://doi.org/10.1542/peds.2018-1771.
20. Brådvik, Louise. "Suicide Risk and Mental Disorders." *International Journal of Environmental Research and Public Health* 15, no. 9 (September 2018): 2028. https://doi.org/10.3390/ijerph15092028.
21. American Association of Suicidology. "American Association of Suicidology Addresses Suicide Rate."
22. Van Orden et al. "Interpersonal Theory of Suicide."
23. Arsenault-Lapierre, Geneviève, Caroline Kim, and Gustavo Turecki. "Psychiatric Diagnoses in 3275 Suicides: A Meta-Analysis." *BMC Psychiatry* 4 (2004):https://doi.org/10.1186/1471-244X-4-37.
24. Humphrey, Nicholas. "The Lure of Death: Suicide and Human Evolution." *Philosophical Transactions of the Royal Society B: Biological Sciences* 373 no. 1754 (September 2018): https://doi.org/10.1098/rstb.2017.0269.
25. Sepp, Tuul. "Suicide Is Unique to Humans and Sets Us Apart from Other Animal Species." Novaator (Estonian Public Broadcasting science news portal), August 2018. https://researchinestonia.eu/2018/08/14/suicide-is-unique-to-humans-and-sets-us-apart-from-other-animal-species/.
26. Buss, David. *Evolutionary Psychology: The New Science of the Mind*. 5th ed. London: Pearson Education, 2014.
27. Dawkins, Richard. *The Selfish Gene*. 2nd ed. Oxford: Oxford University Press, 1989.
28. Nesse, Randolph M. *Good Reasons for Bad Feelings: Insights from the Frontier of Evolutionary Psychiatry*. New York: Dutton, 2019.
29. Humphrey. "Lure of Death."
30. Humphrey.
31. Brink, Andrew. "Depression and Loss: A Theme in Robert Burton's 'Anatomy of Melancholy' (1621)." *Canadian Journal of Psychiatry* 24, no. 8 (December 1979): 767–72. https://doi.org/10.1177/070674377902400811.
32. Tipton, Charles M. "The History of 'Exercise Is Medicine' in Ancient Civilizations." *Advances in Physiology Education* 38, no. 2 (June 2014): 109–17. https://doi.org/10.1152/advan.00136.2013.
33. Humphrey. Lure of Death."

34. Millard, Chris, and Dennis Ougrin. "Narrative Matters: Self-Harm in Britain Post-1945: The Evolution of New Diagnostic Category." *Child and Adolescent Mental Health* 22, no. 3 (July 2017): 175–76. https://doi.org/10.1111/camh.12227.

35. Millard and Ougrin.

36. Mock, Charles N., David C. Grossman, David Mulder, Charles Stewart, and Thomas S. Koepsell. "Health Care Utilization as a Marker for Suicidal Behavior on an American Indian Reservation." *Journal of General Internal Medicine* 11, no. 9 (September 1996): 519–24. https://doi.org/10.1007/bf02599598.

37. Stone, Deborah M., and Alex E. Crosby. "Suicide Prevention: State of the Art Review." *American Journal of Lifestyle Medicine* 8, no. 6 (November/December 2014): 404–20. https://doi.org/10.1177/1559827614551130.

38. Dube, Shanta R., Robert F. Anda, Vincent J. Felitti, Daniel P. Chapman, David F. Williamson, and Wayne H. Giles. "Childhood Abuse, Household Dysfunction, and the Risk of Attempted Suicide throughout the Life Span: Findings from the Adverse Childhood Experiences Study." *Journal of the American Medical Association* 286, no. 24 (2001): 3089. https://doi.org/10.1001/jama.286.24.3089.

39. Shrier, Abigail. *Irreversible Damage: The Transgender Craze Seducing Our Daughters.* Washington, DC: Regnery Publishing, 2020.

40. Wang, Meng-Jie, Kumar Yogeeswaran, Nadia P. Andrews, Diala R. Hawi, and Chris G. Sibley. "How Common Is Cyberbullying among Adults? Exploring Gender, Ethnic, and Age Differences in the Prevalence of Cyberbullying." *Cyberpsychology, Behavior, and Social Networking* 22, no. 11 (November 2019): 736–41. https://doi.org/10.1089/cyber.2019.0146.

41. Czeisler, Mark É., Rashon I. Lane, Emiko Petrosky, Joshua F. Wiley, Aleta Christensen, Rashid Njai, Matthew D. Weaver, Rebecca Robbins, Elise R. Facer-Childs, Laura K. Barger, Charles A. Czeisler, Mark E. Howard, and Shantha M. W. Rajaratnam. "Mental Health, Substance Use, and Suicidal Ideation during the COVID-19 Pandemic—United States, June 24–30, 2020." *Morbidity and Mortality Weekly Report* 69, no. 32 (August 14, 2020): 1049–57. https://doi.org/10.15585/mmwr.mm6932a1.

42. Taylor, Kate. "Gun Sales Boomed in 2020, with Background Checks Hitting Record Highs as Millions of People Bought Guns for the First Time." Business Insider (website), January 15, 2021. https://www.businessinsider.com/gun-sales-boom-2020-background-checks-hit-record-highs-2021-1.

43. Barr, Luke. "Record Number of US Police Officers Died by Suicide in 2019, Advocacy Group Says." ABC News, January 2, 2020. https://abcnews.go.com/Politics/record-number-us-police-officers-died-suicide-2019/story?id=68031484.

44. Gladwell, Malcolm. *Talking to Strangers: What We Should Know about the People We Don't Know.* New York: Back Bay Books, 2019.

45. Wang, Lifei, Yimeng Zhao, Elliot K. Edmiston, Fay Y. Womer, Ran Zhang, Pengfei Zhao, Xiaowei Jiang, Feng Wu, Lingtao Kong, Yifang Zhou, Yanqing Tang, and Shengnan Wei. "Structural and Functional Abnormities of Amygdala and Prefrontal Cortex in Major Depressive Disorder with Suicide Attempts." *Frontiers in Psychiatry* 10 (2019): 923. https://doi.org/10.3389/fpsyt.2019.00923.

46. Swan, Rachel. "Golden Gate Bridge Suicide Nets Delayed Two Years, as People Keep Jumping." *San Francisco Chronicle*, December 12, 2019. https://www.sfchronicle.com/bayarea/article/Golden-Gate-Bridge-suicide-nets-delayed-two-14900278.php.

47. GoldenGateBridgeNet.org. "Saving Lives at the Golden Gate Bridge." Accessed March 1, 2021. https://www.goldengatebridgenet.org.

48. Kling, Arthur. "Effects of Amygdalectomy on Social-Affective Behavior in Non-Human Primates." In *The Neurobiology of the Amygdala*, 511–36. Vol. 2 of *Advances in Behavioral Biology*. Boston: Springer, 1972. https://doi.org/10.1007/978-1-4615-8987-7_18.

49. Nestor, James. *Breath: The New Science of a Lost Art*. New York: Riverhead Books, 2020.

50. Shahtahmasebi, Said. "Examining the Claim That 80-90% of Suicide Cases Had Depression." *Frontiers in Public Health* 1 (December 2013): 62. https://doi.org/10.3389/fpubh.2013.00062.

51. Gurejee, O., B. Oladeji, I. Hwang, W. T. Chiu, R. C. Kessler, N. A. Sampson, J. Alonso, L. H. Andrade, A. Beautrais, G. Borges, E. Bromet, R. Bruffaerts, G. de Girolamo, R. de Graaf, G. Gal, Y. He, C. Hu, N. Iwata, E. G. Karam, V. Kovess-Masféty, H. Matschinger, M. V. Moldovan. J. Posada-Villa, R. Sagar, P. Scocco, S. Seedat, T. Tomoy, and M. K. Nock. "Parental Psychopathology and the Risk of Suicidal Behavior in Their Offspring: Results from the World Mental Health Surveys." *Molecular Psychiatry* 16, no. 12 (December 2011): 1221–33. https://doi.org/10.1038/mp.2010.111.

52. McGuffin, P., A. Marusic, A. Farmer. "What Can Psychiatric Genetics Offer Suicidology?" *Crisis*. 22, no. 2 (2001): 61-65. https://pubmed.ncbi.nlm.nih.gov/11727895/.

53. Voracek, Martin, and Lisa Mariella Loibl. "Genetics of Suicide: A Systematic Review of Twin Studies." *Wiener Klinische Wochenschrift* 119, no. 15–16 (August 2007): 463–75. https://doi.org/10.1007/s00508-007-0823-2.

54. Gurejee et al. "Parental Psychopathology."

55. Franklin, Joseph C., Kathryn R. Fox, Christopher R. Franklin, Evan M. Kleiman, Jessica D. Ribeiro, Adam C. Jaroszewski, Jill M. Hooley, and Matthew K. Nock. "A Brief Mobile App Reduces Nonsuicidal and Suicidal Self-Injury: Evidence from Three Randomized Controlled Trials." *Journal of Consulting and Clinical Psychology* 84, no. 6 (2016): 544–57. https://doi.org/10.1037/ccp0000093.

56. Nock, Matthew K., Jennifer M. Park, Christine T. Finn, Tara L. Deliberto, Halina J. Dour, and Mahzarin R. Banaji. "Measuring the Suicidal Mind: Implicit Cognition Predicts Suicidal Behavior." *Psychological Science* 21, no. 4 (April 2010): 511–17. https://doi.org/10.1177/0956797610364762.

57. Schechner, Sam, and Parmy Olson. "Artificial Intelligence, Facial Recognition Face Curbs in New EU Proposal." *Wall Street Journal*, last modified April 21, 2021. https://www.wsj.com/articles/artificial-intelligence-facial-recognition-face-curbs-in-new-eu-proposal-11619000520.

58. Gladwell, *Talking to Strangers*.

59. Hampson, Neil B. "US Mortality from Carbon Monoxide Poisoning, 1999–2014: Accidental and Intentional Deaths." *Annals of the American Thoracic Society* 13, no. 10 (2016): https://doi.org/10.1513/annalsats.201604-318oc.

CHAPTER 4

1. Kingkade, Tyler, and Elizabeth Chuck. "Suicidal Thoughts Are Increasing in Young Kids, Experts Say. It Began before the Pandemic." NBC News, April 8, 2021. https://www.nbcnews.com/news/us-news/suicidal-thoughts-are-increasing-young -kids-experts-say-it-began-n1263347.

2. Jones, Jason D., Rhonda C. Boyd, Monica E. Calkins, Annisa Ahmed, Tyler M. Moore, Ran Barzilay, Tami D. Benton, and Raquel E. Gur. "Parent-Adolescent Agreement about Adolescents' Suicidal Thoughts." *Pediatrics* 143, no. 2 (February 2019): https://doi.org/10.1542/peds.2018-1771.

3. Bryan, Stierman, Joseph Afful, Margaret Carroll, Chen Te-Ching, Davy Orlando, Steven Fink, and Cheryl Fryar. "National Health and Nutrition Examination Survey 2017–March 2020 Pre-Pandemic Data Files." *National Health Statistics Reports* 158 (June 14, 2021): 1–20. http://dx.doi.org/10.15620/cdc:106273.

4. Rosenberg, M. L., J. C. Smith, L. E. Davidson, and J. M. Conn. "The Emergence of Youth Suicide: An Epidemiologic Analysis and Public Health Perspective." *Annual Review of Public Health* 8, no. 1 (May 1987): 417–40. https://doi.org/10.1146/annurev .pu.08.050187.002221.

5. Carballo, J. J., C. Llorente, L. Kehrmann, I. Flamarique, A. Zuddas, D. Purper-Ouakil, P. J. Hoekstra, D. Coghill, U. M. E. Schulze, R. W. Dittmann, J. K. Buitelaar, J. Castro-Fornieles, K. Lievesley, Paramala Santosh, and C. Arango. "Psychosocial Risk Factors for Suicidality in Children and Adolescents." *European Child & Adolescent Psychiatry* 29, no. 6 (2020): 759–76. https://doi.org/10.1007 /s00787-018-01270-9.

6. National Institute of Mental Health. "Major Depression." Last modified January 2022. https://www.nimh.nih.gov/health/statistics/major-depression.

7. Sheftall, Arielle H., Lindsey Asti, Lisa M. Horowitz, Adrienne Felts, Cynthia A. Fontanella, John V. Campo, and Jeffrey A. Bridge. "Suicide in Elementary School–Aged Children and Early Adolescents." *Pediatrics* 138, no. 4 (October 2016): https: //doi.org/10.1542/peds.2016-0436.

8. Gandhi, Monica, and Jeanne Noble. "The Pandemic's Toll on Teen Mental Health." *Wall Street Journal*, June 10, 2021. https://www.wsj.com/articles/the -pandemics-toll-on-teen-mental-health-11623344542.

9. Xu, Guifeng, Lane Strathearn, Buyun Liu, Binrang Yang, and Wei Bao. "Twenty-Year Trends in Diagnosed Attention-Deficit/Hyperactivity Disorder among US Children and Adolescents, 1997–2016." *JAMA Network Open* 1, no. 4 (2018): https://doi .org/10.1001/jamanetworkopen.2018.1471.

10. Amill-Rosario, Alejandro, Haeyoung Lee, Chengchen Zhang, and Susan dos-Reis. "Psychotropic Prescriptions during the COVID-19 Pandemic Among U.S. Children and Adolescents Receiving Mental Health Services." *Journal of Child and*

Adolescent Psychopharmacology 32, no. 7 (September 2022): 408–14. https://doi.org /10.1089/cap.2022.0037.

11. Guifeng et al. "Twenty-Year Trends in Diagnosed Attention-Deficit/Hyperactivity Disorder."

12. Balaji, Madhumitha, Lakshmi Vijayakumar, Michael Phillips, Smita Panse, Manjeet Santre, Soumitra Pathare, and Vikram Patel. "The Young Lives Matter Study Protocol: A Case-Control Study of the Determinants of Suicide Attempts in Young People in India." *Wellcome Open Research* 5 (2020): 262. https://doi.org/10.12688 /wellcomeopenres.16364.1.

13. Leeb, Rebecca T., Rebecca H. Bitsko, Lakshmi Radhakrishnan, Pedro Martinez, Rashid Njai, and Kristin M. Holland. "Mental Health–Related Emergency Department Visits among Children Aged <18 Years during the COVID-19 Pandemic—United States, January 1–October 17, 2020." *Morbidity and Mortality Weekly Report* 69, no. 45 (November 13, 2020): 1675–80. http://dx.doi.org/10.15585 /mmwr.mm6945a3.

14. American Academy of Child and Adolescent Psychiatry. "Suicide in Children and Teens." Aacap.org, last modified June 2021. https://www.aacap.org/AACAP /Families_and_Youth/Facts_for_Families/FFF-Guide/Teen-Suicide-010.aspx.

15. American Association of Suicidology. "American Association of Suicidology Addresses Suicide Rate During Novel Coronavirus Pandemic," news release, November 2, 2020. https://suicidology.org/2020/11/02/covidandsuicide/.

16. Redfield, Robert. "COVID Webinar Series (Transcript): Robert Redfield, MD." Interview by Kris Rebillot. Buck Institute, July 17, 2020. https://www.buckinstitute .org/covid-webinar-series-transcript-robert-redfield-md/.

17. Zetzsche, Dirk A., and Robera Consiglio. "One Million or One Hundred Million Casualties: The Impact of the COVID-19 Crisis on the Least Developed and Developing Countries." Law Working Paper Series, 2020-008. University of Luxembourg, May 2020. https://doi.org/10.2139/ssrn.3597657.

18. Madhumitha et al. "Young Lives Matter Study Protocol."

19. Charpignon, Marie-Laure, Johnattan Ontiveros, Saahil Sundaresan, Anika Puri, Jay Chandra, Kenneth D. Mandl, and Maimuna Shahnaz Majumder. "Evaluation of Suicides Among US Adolescents during the COVID-19 Pandemic." *JAMA Pediatrics* 176, no. 7 (July 2022): 724–26. https://doi.org/10.1001/jamapediatrics.2022.0515.

20. DeGering, Nicea, and Ian Bartlett. "Bold Plan to Enhance Mental and Behavioral Health Begins in the Intermountain West." ABC4 Utah, October 26, 2020. https: //www.abc4.com/gtu/gtu-sponsor/bold-plan-to-enhance-mental-and-behavioral -health-begins-in-the-intermountain-west/.

21. Brewer, Audrey G., William Doss, Karen M. Sheehan, Matthew M. Davis, and Joseph M. Feinglass. "Trends in Suicidal Ideation-Related Emergency Department Visits for Youth in Illinois: 2016–2021." *Pediatrics* 150, no. 6 (December 2022): https://doi .org/10.1542/peds.2022-056793.

22. Kingkade and Chuck. "Suicidal Thoughts Are Increasing."

23. Janiri, Delfina, Gaelle E. Doucet, Maurizio Pompili, Gabriele Sani, Beatriz Luna, David A. Brent, and Sophia Frangou. "Risk and Protective Factors for Childhood

Suicidality: A US Population-Based Study." *Lancet Psychiatry* 7, no. 4 (April 2020): 317–26. https://doi.org/10.1016/S2215-0366(20)30049-3.

24. Sheftall et al. "Suicide in Elementary School-Aged Children and Early Adolescents."
25. Rabin, Roni Caryn. "U.S. Suicides Declined Over All in 2020 but May Have Risen Among People of Color." *New York Times*, April 15, 2021. https://www.nytimes.com/2021/04/15/health/coronavirus-suicide-cdc.html.
26. Plemmons, Gregory, Matthew Hall, Stephanie Doupnik, James Gay, Charlotte Brown, Whitney Browning, Robert Casey, Katherine Freundlich, David P. Johnson, Carrie Lind, Kris Rehm, Susan Thomas, and Derek Williams. "Hospitalization for Suicide Ideation or Attempt: 2008–2015." *Pediatrics* 141, no. 6 (June 2018): https://doi.org/10.1542/peds.2017-2426.
27. Kingkade and Chuck. "Suicidal Thoughts Are Increasing."
28. Danbeck, Jackson. "Preliminary Autopsy Concludes Kodie Dutcher Died from Pharmacologic Suicide." WMTV—NBC15, July 9, 2020. https://www.nbc15.com/2020/07/09/preliminary-autopsy-concludes-kodie-dutcher-died-from-pharmacologic-suicide/.
29. Kim, Christine. "Orange County Family Shares Teen Suicide Story as Pandemic Warning to Other Parents." NBC Los Angeles, January 19, 2021. https://www.nbclosangeles.com/news/local/orange-county-family-shares-teen-suicide-story-as-pandemic-warning-to-other-parents/2509206/.
30. Burke, Minyvonne. "Maine Teen Dies by Suicide after Struggling to Cope with Pandemic, Father Says." NBC News, December 8, 2020. https://www.nbcnews.com/news/us-news/teen-dies-suicide-after-struggling-cope-pandemic-father-says-n1250442.
31. Encinas, Ciara. "Youth Suicides up in Arizona; Nearly 30% Include Pima County." KGUN 9 Tucson News, November 10, 2020. https://www.kgun9.com/news/local-news/youth-suicides-up-in-arizona-nearly-30-include-pima-county.
32. Hunstable, Brad. "Hayden's Corner—Brad Hunstable on the Tragic Death of His Son Hayden." YouTube, May 1, 2020. Video, 11:11. https://www.youtube.com/watch?v=VJTHFhVyyqI.
33. Green, Erica L. "Surge of Student Suicides Pushes Las Vegas Schools to Reopen." *New York Times*, January 24, 2021. https://www.nytimes.com/2021/01/24/us/politics/student-suicides-nevada-coronavirus.html.
34. Klas. "4th CCSD Suicide Raises Concern of Mental Health Crisis during COVID-19 Pandemic." KLAS. KLAS, November 13, 2020. https://www.8newsnow.com/news/local-news/4th-ccsd-suicide-raises-concern-of-mental-health-crisis-during-covid-19-pandemic/.
35. Klas. "4th CCSD Suicide Raises Concern of Mental Health Crisis during COVID-19 Pandemic."
36. Green, Erica L. "Surge of Student Suicides Pushes Las Vegas Schools to Reopen." *The New York Times*. January 24, 2021. https://www.nytimes.com/2021/01/24/us/politics/student-suicides-nevada-coronavirus.html.
37. Green. "Surge of Student Suicides Pushes Las Vegas Schools to Reopen."
38. Sheftall et al. "Suicide in Elementary School-Aged Children and Early Adolescents."

39. Rabin. "U.S. Suicides Declined Over All."

40. Stierman et al. "National Health and Nutrition Examination Survey."

41. Twenge, Jean M. *IGen: Why Today's Super-Connected Kids Are Growing Up Less Rebellious, More Tolerant, Less Happy—and Completely Unprepared for Adulthood—and What That Means for the Rest of Us.* New York: Atria Books, 2017.

42. Ostic, Dragana, Sikandar Ali Qalati, Belem Barbosa, Syed Mir Muhammad Shah, Esthela Galvan Vela, Ahmed Muhammad Herzallah, and Feng Liu. "Effects of Social Media Use on Psychological Well-Being: A Mediated Model." *Frontiers in Psychology* 12 (June 12, 2021): 678–766. https://doi.org/10.3389/fpsyg.2021.678766.

43. Haidt, Jonathan, and Jean M. Twenge. "This Is Our Chance to Pull Teenagers Out of the Smartphone Trap." *New York Times.* July 31, 2021. https://www.nytimes.com/2021/07/31/opinion/smartphone-iphone-social-media-isolation.html.

44. Twenge, Jean M., and W. Keith Campbell. "Associations between Screen Time and Lower Psychological Well-Being among Children and Adolescents: Evidence from a Population-Based Study." *Preventive Medicine Reports* 12 (December 2018): 271–83. https://doi.org/10.1016/j.pmedr.2018.10.003.

45. Allcott, Hunt, Luca Braghieri, Sarah Eichmeyer, and Matthew Gentzkow. "The Welfare Effects of Social Media." *American Economic Review* 110, no. 3 (March 2020): 629–76. https://doi.org/10.1257/aer.20190658.

46. Sedgwick, Rosemary, Sophie Epstein, Rina Dutta, and Dennis Ougrin. "Social Media, Internet Use and Suicide Attempts in Adolescents." *Current Opinion in Psychiatry* 32, no. 6 (November 2019): 534–41. https://doi.org/10.1097/YCO.0000000000000547.

47. Krause, Adam J., Eti Ben Simon, Bryce A. Mander, Stephanie M. Greer, Jared M. Saletin, Andrea N. Goldstein-Piekarski, and Matthew P. Walker. "The Sleep-Deprived Human Brain." *Nature Reviews Neuroscience* 18, no. 7 (July 2017): 404–18. https://doi.org/10.1038/nrn.2017.55.

48. Twenge and Campbell. "Associations between Screen Time and Lower Psychological Well-Being."

49. Walker, Matthew P., Tiffany Brakefield, Joshua Seidman, Alexandra Morgan, J. Allan Hobson, and Robert Stickgold. "Sleep and the Time Course of Motor Skill Learning." *Learning & Memory* 10, no. 4 (2003): 275–84. https://doi.org/10.1101/lm.58503.

50. Garai, Shuvabrata. "Student Suicides Rising, 28 Lives Lost Every Day." *The Hindu*, January 29, 2020. https://www.thehindu.com/news/national/student-suicides-rising-28-lives-lost-every-day/article61638801.ece.

51. Chatterjee, Rhitu. "Child Psychiatrists Warn That the Pandemic May Be Driving up Kids' Suicide Risk." *NPR.* February 2, 2021. https://www.npr.org/sections/health-shots/2021/02/02/962060105/child-psychiatrists-warn-that-the-pandemic-may-be-driving-up-kids-suicide-risk.

52. Chatterjee. "Child Psychiatrists Warn That the Pandemic May Be Driving Up Kids' Suicide Risk."

53. Hill, Ryan M., Katrina Rufino, Sherin Kurian, Johanna Saxena, Kirti Saxena, and Laurel Williams. "Suicide Ideation and Attempts in a Pediatric Emergency

Department before and during COVID-19." *Pediatrics* 147, no. 3 (March 2021): https://doi.org/10.1542/peds.2020-029280.

54. de Becker, Gavin. *The Gift of Fear: Survival Signals That Protect Us from Violence.* London: Bloomsbury Publishing, 2000.

55. Parikh, Tapan, and John T. Walkup. "The Future of Ketamine in the Treatment of Teen Depression." *American Journal of Psychiatry* 178, no. 4 (April 2021): 288–89. https://doi.org/10.1176/appi.ajp.2020.21020172.

56. Cullen, Kathryn R., Palistha Amatya, Mark G. Roback, Christina Sophia Albott, Melinda Westlund Schreiner, Yanan Ren, Lynn E. Eberly, Patricia Carstedt, Ali Samikoglu, Meredith Gunlicks-Stoessel, Kristina Reigstad, Nathan Horek, Susannah Tye, Kelvin O. Lim, and Bonnie Klimes-Dougan. "Intravenous Ketamine for Adolescents with Treatment-Resistant Depression: An Open-Label Study." *Journal of Child and Adolescent Psychopharmacology* 28, no. 7 (November 2018): 437–44. https://doi.org/10.1089/cap.2018.0030.

57. Weber, Garret, JuHan Yao, Shemeica Binns, and Shinae Namkoong. "Case Report of Subanesthetic Intravenous Ketamine Infusion for the Treatment of Neuropathic Pain and Depression with Suicidal Features in a Pediatric Patient." *Case Reports in Anesthesiology* 2018 (2018): https://doi.org/10.1155/2018/9375910.

58. Kim, Susan, Brittany S. Rush, and Timothy R. Rice. "A Systematic Review of Therapeutic Ketamine Use in Children and Adolescents with Treatment-Resistant Mood Disorders." *European Child & Adolescent Psychiatry* 30, no. 10 (2021): 1485–1501. https://doi.org/10.1007/s00787-020-01542-3.

59. Calabrese, Lori. "Titrated Serial Ketamine Infusions Stop Outpatient Suicidality and Avert ER Visits and Hospitalizations." *International Journal of Psychiatry Research* 2, no. 6 (2019): 1–12. https://doi.org/10.33425/2641-4317.1033.

60. Weber, Yao, Binns, and Namkoong. "Case Report of Subanesthetic Intravenous Ketamine Infusion."

CHAPTER 5

1. Suitt, Thomas Howard. "High Suicide Rates among United States Service Members and Veterans of the Post-9/11 Wars." Costs of War Research Series. Watson Institute for International and Public Affairs, Brown University, June 21, 2021. https://watson.brown.edu/costsofwar/papers/2021/Suicides.

2. America's Warrior Partnership. "Operation Deep Dive Summary of Interim Report." Accessed 2022. https://www.americaswarriorpartnership.org/deep-dive/interview-participants.

3. Lemle, Russell B. "Veterans, Firearms, and Suicide: Safe Storage Prevention Policy and the PREVENTS Roadmap." *Federal Practitioner* 37, no. 9 (September 2020): 426–33. https://doi.org/10.12788/fp.0041.

4. Lee, Michelle Ye Hee. "Hillary Clinton's Misleading Claim That 'Numerous Surveys' Show Veterans Are Satisfied with VA Medical Care." *Washington Post*, November 2, 2015. https://www.washingtonpost.com/news/fact-checker/wp/2015/11/02/hillary-clintons-misleading-claim-that-numerous-surveys-show-veterans-are-satisfied-with-va-medical-care/.

5. US Department of Veterans Affairs. *2019 National Veteran Suicide Prevention Annual Report.* https://www.mentalhealth.va.gov/docs/data-sheets/2019/2019_National _Veteran_Suicide_Prevention_Annual_Report_508.pdf.

6. Lemle. "Veterans, Firearms, and Suicide."

7. Cornum, R., M. D. Matthews, and M. E. P. Seligman. "Comprehensive Soldier Fitness: Building Resilience in a Challenging Institutional Context." *American Psychologist* 66, no. 1 (2011): 4–9. https://doi.org/10.1037/a0021420.

8. Inoue, Catarina, Evan Shawler, Christopher H. Jordan, and Christopher A. Jackson. "Veteran and Military Mental Health Issues." StatPearls (website), January 2022. https://pubmed.ncbi.nlm.nih.gov/34283458/.

9. Warden, Deborah. "Military TBI during the Iraq and Afghanistan Wars." *Journal of Head Trauma Rehabilitation* 21, no. 5 (September 2006): 398–402. https: //doi.org/10.1097/00001199-200609000-00004.

10. Lapierre, Coady B., Andria F. Schwegler, and Bill J. LaBauve. "Posttraumatic Stress and Depression Symptoms in Soldiers Returning from Combat Operations in Iraq and Afghanistan." *Journal of Traumatic Stress* 20, no. 6 (December 2007): 933–43. https://doi.org/10.1002/jts.20278.

11. King, Anthony P., Stefanie R. Block, Rebecca K. Sripada, Sheila Rauch, Nicholas Giardino, Todd Favorite, Michael Angstadt, Daniel Kessler, Robert Welsh, and Israel Liberzon. "Altered Default Mode Network (DMN) Resting State Functional Connectivity Following a Mindfulness-Based Exposure Therapy for Posttraumatic Stress Disorder (PTSD) in Combat Veterans of Afghanistan and Iraq." *Depression and Anxiety* 33, no. 4 (April 2016): 289–99. https://doi.org/10.1002/da.22481.

12. Dregan, Alex, Ann McNeill, Fiona Gaughran, Peter B. Jones, Anna Bazley, Sean Cross, Kate Lillywhite, David Armstrong, Shubulade Smith, David P. J. Osborn, Robert Stewart, Til Wykes, and Matthew Hotopf. "Potential Gains in Life Expectancy from Reducing Amenable Mortality among People Diagnosed with Serious Mental Illness in the United Kingdom." *PLOS One* 15, no. 3 (2020): https://doi.org/10.1371 /journal.pone.0230674.

13. De Hert, Marc, Johan Detraux, and Davy Vancampfort. "The Intriguing Relationship between Coronary Heart Disease and Mental Disorders." *Dialogues in Clinical Neuroscience* 20, no. 1 (2018): 31–40. https://doi.org/10.31887/dcns.2018.20.1 /mdehert.

14. Dennis, Emily L., et al. "Altered White Matter Microstructural Organization in Posttraumatic Stress Disorder across 3047 Adults: Results from the PGC-ENIGMA PTSD Consortium." *Molecular Psychiatry* 26, no. 8 (August 2021): 4315–30. https: //doi.org/10.1038/s41380-019-0631-x.

15. Londoño, Ernesto. "After Six-Decade Hiatus, Experimental Psychedelic Therapy Returns to the V.A." *New York Times.* June 24, 2022. https://www.nytimes .com/2022/06/24/us/politics/psychedelic-therapy-veterans.html.

16. Abdallah, Chadi G., John D. Roache, Lynnette A. Averill, Stacey Young-McCaughan, Brenda Martini, Ralitza Gueorguieva, Timothy Amoroso, Steven M. Southwick, Kevin Guthmiller, Argelio L. López-Roca, Karl Lautenschlager, Jim Mintz, Brett T. Litz, Douglas E. Williamson, Terence M. Keane, Alan L. Peterson,

and John H. Krystal. "Repeated Ketamine Infusions for Antidepressant-Resistant PTSD: Methods of a Multicenter, Randomized, Placebo-Controlled Clinical Trial." *Contemporary Clinical Trials* 81 (June 2019): 11–18. https://doi.org/10.1016/j .cct.2019.04.009.

17. Feder, Adriana, Sara Costi, Sarah B. Rutter, Abigail B. Collins, Usha Govindarajulu, Manish K. Jha, Sarah R. Horn, Marin Kautz, Morgan Corniquel, Katherine A. Collins, Laura Bevilacqua, Andrew M. Glasgow, Jess Brallier, Robert H. Pietrzak, James W. Murrough, and Dennis Charney. "A Randomized Controlled Trial of Repeated Ketamine Administration for Chronic Posttraumatic Stress Disorder." *American Journal of Psychiatry* 178, no. 2 (February 2021): 193–202. https://doi .org/10.1176/appi.ajp.2020.20050596.

18. McGhee, Laura L., Christopher V. Maani, Thomas H. Garza, Terry M. Slater, Lawrence N. Petz, and Marcie Fowler. "The Intraoperative Administration of Ketamine to Burned US. Service Members Does Not Increase the Incidence of Post-Traumatic Stress Disorder." Supplement, *Military Medicine* 179, no. 8S (August 2014): 41–46. https://doi.org/10.7205/milmed-d-13-00481.

19. McGhee, Laura L., Christopher V. Maani, Thomas H. Garza, Kathryn M. Gaylord, and Ian H. Black. "The Correlation between Ketamine and Posttraumatic Stress Disorder in Burned Service Members." Supplement, *Journal of Trauma* 64, no. 2 (February 2008): S195–99. https://doi.org/10.1097/TA.0b013e318160ba1d.

20. Pradhan, Basant, Ludmil Mitrev, Ruin Moaddell, and Irving W. Wainer. "D-Serine Is a Potential Biomarker for Clinical Response in Treatment of Post-Traumatic Stress Disorder Using (R,S)-Ketamine Infusion and TIMBER Psychotherapy: A Pilot Study." *Biochimica et Biophysica Acta—Proteins and Proteomics* 1866, no. 7 (July 2018): 831–39. https://doi.org/10.1016/j.bbapap.2018.03.006.

21. Pradhan, Mitrev, Moaddell, and Wainer.

22. Krystal, John H., Chadi G. Abdallah, Gerard Sanacora, Dennis S. Charney, and Ronald S. Duman. "Ketamine: A Paradigm Shift for Depression Research and Treatment." *Neuron* 101, no. 5 (2019): 774–78. https://doi.org/10.1016/j .neuron.2019.02.005.

23. Bryan, Craig J., M. David Rudd, and Evelyn Wertenberger. "Reasons for Suicide Attempts in a Clinical Sample of Active Duty Soldiers." *Journal of Affective Disorders* 144, no. 1–2 (January 2013): 148–52. https://doi.org/10.1016/j.jad.2012.06.030.

24. Suitt. "High Suicide Rates."

25. Kalmoe, Molly C., Matthew B. Chapman, Jessica A. Gold, and Andrea M. Giedinghagen. "Physician Suicide: A Call to Action." *Missouri Medicine* 116, no. 3 (May-June 2019): 211–16. https://www.ncbi.nlm.nih.gov/pmc/articles/PMC6690303/.

26. Knoll, Corina, Ali Watkins, and Michael Rothfeld. "'I Couldn't Do Anything': The Virus and an E.R. Doctor's Suicide." *New York Times*, July 11, 2020. https://www .nytimes.com/2020/07/11/nyregion/lorna-breen-suicide-coronavirus.html.

27. Wang, Amy B. "Another Sheriff's Deputy Dies by Suicide. This Time, His Boss Wants People to Talk about It." *Washington Post*. August 2, 2017. https://www .washingtonpost.com/news/post-nation/wp/2017/08/02/another-sheriffs-deputy -commits-suicide-his-boss-wants-people-to-talk-about-it-this-time/.

28. O'Hara, Andrew F., John M. Violanti, Richard L. Levenson Jr., and Ronald G. Clark Sr. "National Police Suicide Estimates: Web Surveillance Study III." *International Journal of Emergency Mental Health* 15, no. 1 (2013): 31–38. https://pubmed.ncbi.nlm.nih.gov/24187885/.

29. Police Executive Research Forum. *An Occupational Risk: What Every Police Agency Should Do to Prevent Suicide Among Its Officers.* Critical Issues in Policing Series. Washington, DC: Police Executive Research Forum, October 2019. https://www.policeforum.org/assets/PreventOfficerSuicide.pdf.

30. O'Hara et al. "National Police Suicide Estimates."

31. Police Executive Research Forum. *An Occupational Risk.*

32. Hermann, Peter. "Two Police Officers Who Helped Fight the Capitol Mob Have Died of Suicide. Many More Are Hurting." *Philadelphia Inquirer*, February 12, 2021. https://www.inquirer.com/news/nation-world/capitol-attack-police-suicides-jeffrey -smith-howard-liebengood-20210212.html.

33. Hermann.

34. Solender, Andrew. "Fourth Police Officer Who Responded to Capitol Riot Dies by Suicide." *Forbes*, August 3, 2021. https://www.forbes.com/sites/andrewsolender /2021/08/03/fourth-police-officer-who-responded-to-capitol-riot-dies-by-suicide/.

CHAPTER 6

1. Sussman, Steve, and Alan N. Sussman. "Considering the Definition of Addiction." *International Journal of Environmental Research and Public Health* 8, no. 10 (October 2011): 4025–38. https://doi.org/10.3390/ijerph8104025.

2. CDC National Center for Health Statistics. *Drug Overdose Deaths in the United States, 2001–2021.* NHCS Data Brief No. 457, December 2022. https://www.cdc .gov/nchs/products/databriefs/db457.htm.

3. Montana Department of Justice. "AG Knudsen: New Data Show Fentanyl Is Top Public Safety Threat in Montana." DOJMT.gov, August 16, 2022. https://dojmt.gov/ ag-knudsen-new-data-show-fentanyl-is-top-public-safety-threat-in-montana/.

4. Nordic Medico-Statistical Committee. *Drug Related Deaths in the Nordic Countries—Revision of the Statistical Definition.* Copenhagen: Nordic Medico -Statistical Committee, 2017. https://norden.diva-portal.org/smash/get/diva2:1170945 /FULLTEXT01.pdf.

5. Lovett, Ian. "Fentanyl Has Spread West and Overdoses Are Surging." *Wall Street Journal*, April 15, 2021. https://www.wsj.com/articles/fentanyl-has-spread-west-and -overdoses-are-surging-11618484400.

6. Weiner, Stacy. "COVID-19 and the Opioid Crisis: When a Pandemic and an Epidemic Collide." Association of American Medical Colleges, July 27, 2020. https://www.aamc.org/news-insights/covid-19-and-opioid-crisis-when-pandemic -and-epidemic-collide.

7. Schiller, Elizabeth Y., Amandeep Goyal, and Oren J. Mechanic. "Opioid Overdose." StatPearls (website), 2022. https://www.ncbi.nlm.nih.gov/books/NBK470415/.

8. Lovett. "Fentanyl Has Spread West."

9. CDC National Center for Health Statistics. *Drug Overdose Deaths in the United States.*

Endnotes

10. Selsky, Andrew. "Mixed Results for Oregon's Pioneering Drug Decriminalization." Associated Press, April 3, 2022. https://apnews.com/article/health-business-europe -oregon-salem-158728e57e1d48bc957c5b907bcda5f5.

11. Dubey, Mahua Jana, Ritwik Ghosh, Subham Chatterjee, Payel Biswas, Subhankar Chatterjee, and Souvik Dubey. "COVID-19 and Addiction." *Diabetes & Metabolic Syndrome* 14, no. 5 (September-October 2020): 817–23. https://doi .org/10.1016/j.dsx.2020.06.008.

12. Gage, Suzanne H., and Harry R. Sumnall. "Rat Park: How a Rat Paradise Changed the Narrative of Addiction." *Addiction* 114, no. 5 (May 2019): 917–22. https://doi .org/10.1111/add.14481.

13. Weiner. "COVID-19 and the Opioid Crisis."

14. Maté, Gabor, and Daniel Maté. *The Myth of Normal: Trauma, Illness, and Healing in a Toxic Culture.* New York: Penguin Young Readers, 2022.

15. Joseph, Jay. *The Trouble with Twin Studies: A Reassessment of Twin Research in the Social and Behavioral Sciences.* New York: Routledge, 2016.

16. Kaskutas, Lee Ann. "Alcoholics Anonymous Effectiveness: Faith Meets Science." *Journal of Addictive Diseases* 28, no. 2 (2009): 145–57. https://doi.org /10.1080/10550880902772464.

17. Moles, Anna, Brigitte L. Kieffer, and Francesca R. D'Amato. "Deficit in Attachment Behavior in Mice Lacking the μ-Opioid Receptor Gene." *Science* 304, no. 5679 (June 25, 2004): 1983–86. https://doi.org/10.1126/science.1095943.

18. Stanley, Barbara, Leo Sher, Scott Wilson, Rolf Ekman, Yung-Yu Huang, and J. John Mann. "Non-Suicidal Self-Injurious Behavior, Endogenous Opioids and Monoamine Neurotransmitters." *Journal of Affective Disorders* 124, no. 1–2 (July 2010): 134–40. https://doi.org/10.1016/j.jad.2009.10.028.

19. Krupitsky, Evgeny, Andrey Burakov, Tatyana Romanova, Igor Dunaevsky, Rick Strassman, and Alexander Grinenko. "Ketamine Psychotherapy for Heroin Addiction: Immediate Effects and Two-Year Follow-Up." *Journal of Substance Abuse Treatment* 23, no. 4 (December 2002): 273–83. https://doi.org/10.1016/s0740-5472(02)00275-1.

20. Straussner, Shulamith, Lala Ashenberg, and Alexandrea Josephine Calnan. "Trauma through the Life Cycle: A Review of Current Literature." *Clinical Social Work Journal* 42, no. 4 (December 2014): 323–35. https://doi.org/10.1007/s10615 -014-0496-z.

21. Straussner, Ashenberg, and Calnan.

22. McAndrew, Amy, Will Lawn, Tobias Stevens, Lilla Porffy, Brigitta Brandner, and Celia J. A. Morgan. "A Proof-of-Concept Investigation into Ketamine as a Pharmacological Treatment for Alcohol Dependence: Study Protocol for a Randomised Controlled Trial." *Trials* 18, no. 1 (2017): https://doi.org/10.1186/s13063-017-1895-6.

23. Wolfson, Phil, and Glenn Hartelius. *The Ketamine Papers: Science, Therapy, and Transformation.* Santa Cruz, CA: Multidisciplinary Association for Psychedelic Studies, 2016.

24. Wolfson and Hartelius.

25. Krupitsky, E. M., and A. Y. Grinenko. "Ketamine Psychedelic Therapy (KPT): A Review of the Results of Ten Years of Research." *Journal of Psychoactive Drugs* 29, no. 2 (1997): 165–83. https://doi.org/10.1080/02791072.1997.10400185.

26. Grabski, Meryem, Amy McAndrew, Will Lawn, Beth Marsh, Laura Raymen, Tobias Stevens, Lorna Hardy, Fiona Warren, Michael Bloomfield, Anya Borissova, Emily Maschauer, Rupert Broomby, Robert Price, Rachel Coathup, David Gilhooly, Edward Palmer, Richard Gordon-Williams, Robert Hill, Jen Harris, O. Merve Mollaahmetoglu, Valerie Curran, Brigitta Bradner, Anne Lingford-Hughes, and Celia J. A. Morgan. "Adjunctive Ketamine with Relapse Prevention–Based Psychological Therapy in the Treatment of Alcohol Use Disorder." *American Journal of Psychiatry* 179, no. 2 (2022): 152–62. https://doi.org/10.1176/appi.ajp.2021.21030277.

27. Kaskutas. "Alcoholics Anonymous Effectiveness."

28. Mills, I. H., G. R. Park, A. R. Manara, and R. J. Merriman. "Treatment of Compulsive Behaviour in Eating Disorders with Intermittent Ketamine Infusions." *QJM: An International Journal of Medicine* 91, no. 7 (July 1998): 493–503. https://doi.org/10.1093/qjmed/91.7.493.

29. Scolnick, Barbara, Beth Zupec-Kania, Lori Calabrese, Chiye Aoki, and Thomas Hildebrandt. "Remission from Chronic Anorexia Nervosa with Ketogenic Diet and Ketamine: Case Report." *Frontiers in Psychiatry* 11 (July 2020): https://doi.org/10.3389/fpsyt.2020.00763.

30. Beckwith, Caroline. "How I Got out of Anorexia." YouTube, August 8, 2020. Video, 22:31. https://www.youtube.com/watch?v=U9fcyhukwbI.

CHAPTER 7

1. Fagan, Kate. *What Made Maddy Run: The Secret Struggles and Tragic Death of an All-American Teen.* New York: Back Bay Books, 2017.

2. Calfas, Jennifer. "A New Death Shakes a Campus Rattled by Student Suicides." *Wall Street Journal*, October 1, 2019. https://www.wsj.com/articles/a-new-death-shakes-a-campus-rattled-by-student-suicides-11569861012.

3. Calfas. "A New Death Shakes a Campus Rattled by Student Suicides."

4. Mofatteh, Mohammad. "Risk Factors Associated with Stress, Anxiety, and Depression among University Undergraduate Students." *AIMS Public Health* 8, no. 1 (December 25, 2021): 36–65. https://doi.org/10.3934/publichealth.2021004. PMID: 33575406; PMCID: PMC7870388.

5. Zivin, Kara, Daniel Eisenberg, Sarah E. Gollust, and Ezra Golberstein. "Persistence of Mental Health Problems and Needs in a College Student Population." *Journal of Affective Disorders* 117, no. 3 (October 2009: 180–85. https://doi.org/10.1016/j.jad.2009.01.001.

6. Rao, Ashwin L., Irfan M. Asif, Jonathan A. Drezner, Brett G. Toresdahl, and Kimberly G. Harmon. "Suicide in National Collegiate Athletic Association (NCAA) Athletes: A 9-Year Analysis of the NCAA Resolutions Database." *Sports Health* 7, no. 5 (2015): 452–57. https://doi.org/10.1177/1941738115587675.

7. Fagan. *What Made Maddy Run.*

8. Twenge, Jean M., Jonathan Haidt, Andrew B. Blake, Cooper McAllister, Hannah Lemon, and Astrid Le Roy. "Worldwide Increases in Adolescent Loneliness." *Journal of Adolescence* 93, no. 1 (December 2021): 257–69. https://doi.org/10.1016/j .adolescence.2021.06.006.

9. Seltzer, Leslie J., Ashley R. Prososki, Toni E. Ziegler, and Seth D. Pollak. "Instant Messages vs. Speech: Hormones and Why We Still Need to Hear Each Other." *Evolution and Human Behavior* 33, no. 1 (January 2012): 42-45. https://doi .org/10.1016/j.evolhumbehav.2011.05.004.

10. Mofatteh. "Risk Factors Associated with Stress."

11. Drew Robinson, in discussion with the author, April 2020.

12. Passan, Jeff. "San Francisco Giants Outfielder Drew Robinson's Remarkable Second Act." ESPN.com, last updated May 11, 2021. https://www.espn.com/mlb/story/_/ id/30800732/san-francisco-giants-outfielder- drew-robinson-remarkable-second-act.

13. Clemmons, Anna Katherine. "Pushed by Players, the N.F.L. Works to Embrace Mental Health." *New York Times*, November 26, 2021. https://www.nytimes.com /2021/11/26/sports/football/nfl-mental-health.html.

14. Osaka, Naomi. "It's O.K. Not to Be O.K." *Time*, July 8, 2021.

15. Thomas, Louisa. "A Year That Changed How Athletes Think about Mental Health." *New Yorker*, December 20, 2021. https://www.newyorker.com/culture /2021-in-review/a-year-that changed how-athletes-think-about-mental-health.

16. Darren Waller, in discussion with the author, 2023.

17. Haridy, Rich. "Performance-Enhancing Psychedelics: Can LSD Make You Better at Sport?" New Atlas (website), July 20, 2021. https://newatlas.com/sports /performance-enhancing-psychedelics-lsd-olympics-sport-microdosing/.

18. Oroc, James. "Psychedelics and Extreme Sports." *MAPS Bulletin*, vol. 21, no. 1, accessed January 8, 2023. https://maps.org/news-letters/v21n1/v21n1-25to29.pdf.

19. Miesha Tate, in discussion with the author, 2023.

20. McGuffin, Peter, Andrej Marušič, and Anne Farmer. "What Can Psychiatric Genetics Offer Suicidology?" *Crisis* 22, no. 2 (2001): 61–65. https://doi.org/10.1027 /0227-5910.22.2.61.

21. Siebert, Amanda. "13 Professional Athletes Who Have Used Psychedelics." The Dales Report (website), December 16, 2021. https://thedalesreport.com /psychedelics/13-professional-athletes-who-have-used-psychedelics/.

22. *Real Sports with Bryant Gumbel*. Season 26, episode 10, "Psychedelic Drugs to Treat Head Injuries." Aired November 24, 2020, on HBO. https://www.imdb.com/title /tt13310420/?ref_=ttep_ep10.

23. Bleier, Evan. "NFL Day-Tripper Kenny Stills Is Embracing the Healing Power of Using Psychedelics." InsideHook (website), April 21, 2022. https://www.insidehook .com/article/sports/nfl-kenny-stills-healing-power-psychedelics.

CHAPTER 8

1. National Institute of Mental Health. "Major Depression." Last modified January 2022. https://www.nimh.nih.gov/health/statistics/major-depression.

2. Mann, J. John, Christina A. Michel, and Randy P. Auerbach. "Improving Suicide Prevention through Evidence-Based Strategies: A Systematic Review." *American Journal of Psychiatry* 178, no. 7 (July 2021): 611–24. https://doi.org/10.1176/appi .ajp.2020.20060864.

3. D'Anci, Kristen E., Stacey Uhl, Gina Giradi, and Constance Martin. "Treatments for the Prevention and Management of Suicide: A Systematic Review." *Annals of Internal Medicine* 171, no. 5 (August 27, 2019): 334–42. https://doi .org/10.7326/m19-0869.

4. Brown, Gregory K., Thomas Ten Have, Gregg R. Henriques, Sharon X. Xie, Judd E. Hollander, and Aaron T. Beck. "Cognitive Therapy for the Prevention of Suicide Attempts." *Journal of the American Medical Association* 294, no. 5 (2005): 563–70. https://doi.org/10.1001/jama.294.5.563.

5. Oaklander, Mandy. "Depression: Doctors Are Turning to Ketamine for Treatment." *Time*, July 27, 2017. https://time.com/4876098/new-hope-for-depression/.

6. Harmer, Bonnie, Sarah Lee, and Truc vi H. Duong. "Suicidal Ideation." StatPearls (website), 2022. https://www.ncbi.nlm.nih.gov/books/NBK565877/.

7. Oaklander. "Depression: Doctors Are Turning to Ketamine."

8. Hillhouse, Todd M., and Joseph H. Porter. "A Brief History of the Development of Antidepressant Drugs: From Monoamines to Glutamate." *Experimental and Clinical Psychopharmacology* 23, no. 1 (February 23, 2015): 1–21. https://doi.org/10.1037 /a0038550.

9. Thomas Insel, in discussion with the author, 2022.

10. Phillips, Jennifer L., Sandhaya Norris, Jeanne Talbot, Taylor Hatchard, Abigail Ortiz, Meagan Birmingham, Olabisi Owoeye, Lisa A. Batten, and Pierre Blier. "Single and Repeated Ketamine Infusions for Reduction of Suicidal Ideation in Treatment-Resistant Depression." *Neuropsychopharmacology* 45 (March 2020): 606–12. https: //doi.org/10.1038/s41386-019-0570-x.

11. Can, Adem T., Daniel F. Hermens, Megan Dutton, Cyrana C. Gallay, Emma Jensen, Monique Jones, Jennifer Scherman, Denise A. Beaudequin, Cian Yang, Paul E. Schwenn, and Jim Lagopoulos. "Low Dose Oral Ketamine Treatment in Chronic Suicidality: An Open-Label Pilot Study." *Translational Psychiatry* 11, no. 1 (February 2021): https://doi.org/10.1038/s41398-021-01230-z.

12. Maltbie, Eric A., Gopinath S. Kaundinya, and Leonard L. Howell. "Ketamine and Pharmacological Imaging: Use of Functional Magnetic Resonance Imaging to Evaluate Mechanisms of Action." *Behavioural Pharmacology* 28, no. 8 (2017): 610–22. https://doi.org/10.1097/fbp.0000000000000354.

13. Wu, Hao, Neil K. Savalia, and Alex C. Kwan. "Ketamine for a Boost of Neural Plasticity: How, but Also When?" *Biological Psychiatry* 89, no. 11 (June 2021): 1030–32. https://doi.org/10.1016/j.biopsych.2021.03.014.

14. Calabrese, Lori. "Titrated Serial Ketamine Infusions Stop Outpatient Suicidality and Avert ER Visits and Hospitalizations." *International Journal of Psychiatry Research* 2, no. 6 (2019): 1–12. https://doi.org/10.33425/2641-4317.1033.

15. Ballard, Elizabeth D., Dawn F. Ionescu, Jennifer L. Vande Voort, Mark J. Niciu, Erica M. Richards, David A. Luckenbaugh, Nancy E. Brutsché, Rezvan Ameli,

Maura L. Furey, and Carlos A. Zarate Jr. "Improvement in Suicidal Ideation after Ketamine Infusion: Relationship to Reductions in Depression and Anxiety." *Journal of Psychiatric Research* 58 (November 2014): 161–66. https://doi.org/10.1016/j .jpsychires.2014.07.027.

16. Price, Rebecca B., Matthew K. Nock, Dennis S. Charney, and Sanjay J. Mathew. "Effects of Intravenous Ketamine on Explicit and Implicit Measures of Suicidality in Treatment-Resistant Depression." *Biological Psychiatry* 66, no. 5 (September 2009): 522–26. https://doi.org/10.1016/j.biopsych.2009.04.029.

17. Can et al. "Low Dose Oral Ketamine Treatment."

18. Dockrill, Peter. "Oral Ketamine Experiment Reduces Suicidal Thoughts in over Two-Thirds of Patients." ScienceAlert, February 9, 2021. https://www.sciencealert.com /oral-ketamine-experiment-reduces-suicidal-thoughts-in-over-two-thirds-of-patients.

19. Grande, Lucinda A. "Sublingual Ketamine for Rapid Relief of Suicidal Ideation." *Primary Care Companion for CNS Disorders* 19, no. 2 (2017): https://doi.org/10.4088 /pcc.16l02012.

20. Loveday, Brighton A., and Jill Sindt. "Ketamine Protocol for Palliative Care in Cancer Patients with Refractory Pain." *Journal of the Advanced Practitioner in Oncology* 6, no. 6 (November 1, 2015): 555–61. https://doi.org/10.6004/jadpro.6.6.4.

21. Fan, Wei, HaiKou Yang, Yong Sun, Jun Zhang, Guangming Li, Ying Zheng, and Yi Liu. "Ketamine Rapidly Relieves Acute Suicidal Ideation in Cancer Patients: A Randomized Controlled Clinical Trial." *Oncotarget* 8, no. 2 (January 10, 2017): 2356–60. https://doi.org/10.18632/oncotarget.13743.

22. Olfson, Mark, Y. Nina Gao, Ming Xie, Sara Wiesel Cullen, and Steven C. Marcus. "Suicide Risk among Adults with Mental Health Emergency Department Visits with and without Suicidal Symptoms." *Journal of Clinical Psychiatry* 82, no. 6 (2021): https://doi.org/10.4088/jcp.20m13833.

23. Insel, Thomas R. *Healing: Our Path from Mental Illness to Mental Health.* New York: Penguin Press, 2022.

24. Larkin, Gregory Luke, and Annette L. Beautrais. "A Preliminary Naturalistic Study of Low-Dose Ketamine for Depression and Suicide Ideation in the Emergency Department." *International Journal of Neuropsychopharmacology* 14, no. 8 (September 2011): 1127–31. https://doi.org/10.1017/s1461145711000629.

25. Domany, Yoav, Richard C. Shelton, and Cheryl B. McCullumsmith. "Ketamine for Acute Suicidal Ideation. An Emergency Department Intervention: A Randomized, Double-Blind, Placebo-Controlled, Proof-of-Concept Trial." *Depression and Anxiety* 37, no. 3 (March 2020): 224–33. https://doi.org/10.1002/da.22975.

26. Lindahl, V., J. L. Pearson, and L. Colpe. "Prevalence of Suicidality during Pregnancy and the Postpartum." *Archives of Women's Mental Health* 8, no. 2 (June 2005): 77–87. https://doi.org/10.1007/s00737-005-0080-1.

27. Hansotte, Elinor, Shirley I. Payne, and Suzanne M. Babich. "Positive Postpartum Depression Screening Practices and Subsequent Mental Health Treatment for Low-Income Women in Western Countries: A Systematic Literature Review." *Public Health Reviews* 38, no. 1 (2017): https://doi.org/10.1186/s40985-017-0050-y.

28. Ma, Jia-Hui, Sai-Ying Wang, He-Ya Yu, Dan-Yang Li, Shi-Chao Luo, Shan-Shan Zheng, Li-Fei Wan, and Kai-Ming Duan. "Prophylactic Use of Ketamine Reduces Postpartum Depression in Chinese Women Undergoing Cesarean Section." *Psychiatry Research* 279 (September 2019): 252–58. https://doi.org/10.1016/j.psychres .2019.03.026.

29. Hansotte, Payne, and Babich. "Positive Postpartum Depression Screening Practices."

30. Ma et al. "Prophylactic Use of Ketamine."

31. Guglielminotti, Jean, and Guohua Li. "Exposure to General Anesthesia for Cesarean Delivery and Odds of Severe Postpartum Depression Requiring Hospitalization." *Anesthesia & Analgesia* 131, no. 5 (November 2020): 1421–29. https://doi.org/10.1213/ ane.0000000000004663.

32. Cavalli, Eugenio, Santa Mammana, Ferdinando Nicoletti, Placido Bramanti, and Emanuela Mazzon. "The Neuropathic Pain: An Overview of the Current Treatment and Future Therapeutic Approaches." *International Journal of Immunopathology and Pharmacology* 33 (2019): https://doi.org/10.1177/2058738419838383.

33. Shanthanna, Harsha, Medha Huilgol, and Vinay Kumar Manivackam. "Early and Effective Use of Ketamine for Treatment of Phantom Limb Pain." *Indian Journal of Anaesthesia* 54, no. 2 (March-April 2010): 157–59. https://doi.org /10.4103/0019-5049.63632.

34. Haroon, Ebrahim, and Andrew H. Miller. "Inflammation Effects on Brain Glutamate in Depression: Mechanistic Considerations and Treatment Implications." *Current Topics in Behavioral Neurosciences* 31 (2017): 173–98. https://doi.org/10.1007 /7854_2016_40.

35. Zhou, W., N. Wang, C. Yang, X.-M. Li, Z.-Q. Zhou, and J.-J. Yang. "Ketamine-Induced Antidepressant Effects Are Associated with AMPA Receptors-Mediated Upregulation of mTOR and BDNF in Rat Hippocampus and Prefrontal Cortex." *European Psychiatry* 29, no. 7 (September 2014): 419–23. https://doi.org/10.1016/j .eurpsy.2013.10.005.

36. Collo, Ginetta, and Emilio Merlo Pich. "Ketamine Enhances Structural Plasticity in Human Dopaminergic Neurons: Possible Relevance for Treatment-Resistant Depression." *Neural Regeneration Research* 13, no. 4 (April 2018): 645–46. https:// doi.org/10.4103/1673-5374.230288.

37. de Vos, Cato M., Natasha L. Mason, and Kim P. Kuypers. "Psychedelics and Neuroplasticity: A Systematic Review Unraveling the Biological Underpinnings of Psychedelics." *Frontiers in Psychiatry* 12 (September 10, 2021). https://doi.org/10.3389 /fpsyt.2021.724606. PMID: 34566723; PMCID: PMC8461007.

38. Ding, Y., N. Lawrence, E. Olié, F. Cyprien, E. le Bars, A. Bonafé, M. L. Phillips, P. Courtet, and F. Jollant. "Prefrontal Cortex Markers of Suicidal Vulnerability in Mood Disorders: A Model-Based Structural Neuroimaging Study with a Translational Perspective." *Translational Psychiatry* 5, no. 2 (February 2015): https: //doi.org/10.1038/tp.2015.1.

39. Pirnia, T., S. H. Joshi, A. M. Leaver, M. Vasavada, S. Njau, R. P. Woods, R. Espinoza, and K. L. Narr. "Electroconvulsive Therapy and Structural Neuroplasticity in

Neocortical, Limbic and Paralimbic Cortex." *Translational Psychiatry* 6, no. 6 (June 2016): https://doi.org/10.1038/tp.2016.102.

40. Phoumthipphavong, Victoria, Florent Barthas, Samantha Hassett, and Alex C. Kwan. "Longitudinal Effects of Ketamine on Dendritic Architecture *In Vivo* in the Mouse Medial Frontal Cortex." *eNeuro* 3, no. 2 (March 2016): https://doi.org/10.1523/eneuro.0133-15.2016.

41. Maltbie, Eric, Kaundinya Gopinath, Naoko Urushino, Doty Kempf, and Leonard Howell. "Ketamine-Induced Brain Activation in Awake Female Nonhuman Primates: A Translational Functional Imaging Model." *Psychopharmacology* 233 (October 2016): 961–72. https://doi.org/10.1007/s00213-015-4175-8.

42. Williams, Nolan R., Boris D. Heifets, Christine Blasey, Keith Sudheimer, Jaspreet Pannu, Heather Pankow, Jessica Hawkins, Justin Birnbaum, David Lyons, Carolyn I. Rodriguez, and Alan F. Schatzberg. "Attenuation of Antidepressant Effects of Ketamine by Opioid Receptor Antagonism." *American Journal of Psychiatry* 175, no. 12 (December 2018): 1205–15. https://doi.org/10.1176/appi.ajp.2018.18020138.

43. Yoon, Gihyun, Ismene L. Petrakis, and John H. Krystal. "Association of Combined Naltrexone and Ketamine with Depressive Symptoms in a Case Series of Patients with Depression and Alcohol Use Disorder." *JAMA Psychiatry* 76, no. 3 (2019): 337–38. https://doi.org/10.1001/jamapsychiatry.2018.3990.

44. Ristevska-Dimitrovska, Gordana, Rinaldo Shishkov, Vesna Pejoska Gerazova, Viktorija Vujovik, Branislav Stefanovski, Antoni Novotni, Petar Marinov, and Izabela Filov. "Different Serum BDNF Levels in Depression: Results from BDNF Studies in FYR Macedonia and Bulgaria." *Psychiatria Danubina* 25, no. 2 (June 2013): 123–27. https://pubmed.ncbi.nlm.nih.gov/23793275/.

45. Zhou et al. "Ketamine-Induced Antidepressant Effects."

46. Miao, Zhuang, Yan Wang, and Zhongsheng Sun. "The Relationships between Stress, Mental Disorders, and Epigenetic Regulation of BDNF." *International Journal of Molecular Sciences* 21, no. 4 (February 18, 2020): 1375. https://doi.org/10.3390/ijms21041375.

47. Zhang, Xuemei, Yinglian Zhou, Hulun Li, Rui Wang, Dan Yang, Bing Li, and Jin Fu. "Intravenous Administration of DPSCs and BDNF Improves Neurological Performance in Rats with Focal Cerebral Ischemia." *International Journal of Molecular Medicine* 41 (February 28, 2018): 3185–94. https://doi.org/10.3892/ijmm.2018.3517.

48. Wang, Nan, Hai-Ying Yu, Xiao-Feng Shen, Zhi-Qin Gao, Chun Yang, Jian-Jun Yang, and Guang-Fen Zhang. "The Rapid Antidepressant Effect of Ketamine in Rats Is Associated with Down-Regulation of Pro-Inflammatory Cytokines in the Hippocampus." *Upsala Journal of Medical Sciences* 120, no. 4 (2015): 241–48. https://doi.org/10.3109/03009734.2015.1060281.

49. Binder, Devin K., and Helen E. Scharfman. "Mini Review." *Growth Factors* 22, no. 3 (September 2004): 123–31. https://doi.org/10.1080/08977190410001723308.

50. Eisen, Rebecca B., Stefan Perera, Monica Bawor, Brittany B. Dennis, Wala El-Sheikh, Jane DeJesus, Sumathy Rangarajan, Judith Vair, Heather Sholer, Nicole Hutchinson, Elizabeth Iordan, Pam Mackie, Shofiqul Islam, Mahshid Dehghan, Jennifer Brasch, Rebecca Anglin, Luciano Minuzzi, Lehana Thabane, and Zainab Samaan. "Exploring

the Association between Serum BDNF and Attempted Suicide." *Scientific Reports* 6 (2016): https://doi.org/10.1038/srep25229.

51. Hashimoto, Kenji. "Role of the mTOR Signaling Pathway in the Rapid Antidepressant Action of Ketamine." *Expert Review of Neurotherapeutics* 11, no. 1 (2011): 33–36. https://doi.org/10.1586/ern.10.176.

52. Steiner, Johann, Hendrik Bielau, Ralf Brisch, Peter Danos, Oliver Ullrich, Christian Mawrin, Hans-Gert Bernstein, and Bernhard Bogerts. "Immunological Aspects in the Neurobiology of Suicide: Elevated Microglial Density in Schizophrenia and Depression Is Associated with Suicide." *Journal of Psychiatric Research* 42, no. 2 (January 2008): 151–57. https://doi.org/10.1016/j.jpsychires.2006.10.013.

53. Raison, Charles L., Andrey S. Borisov, Matthias Majer, Daniel F. Drake, Giuseppe Pagnoni, Bobbi J. Woolwine, Gerald J. Vogt, Breanne Massung, and Andrew H. Miller. "Activation of Central Nervous System Inflammatory Pathways by Interferon-Alpha: Relationship to Monoamines and Depression." *Biological Psychiatry* 65, no. 4 (2009): 296–303. https://doi.org/10.1016/j.biopsych.2008.08.010.

54. Choudhury, Divya, Anita E. Autry, Kimberley F. Tolias, and Vaishnav Krishnan. "Ketamine: Neuroprotective or Neurotoxic?" *Frontiers in Neuroscience* 15 (September 10, 2021): https://doi.org/10.3389/fnins.2021.672526.

55. Pribish, Abby, Nicole Wood, and Arun Kalava. "A Review of Nonanesthetic Uses of Ketamine." *Anesthesiology Research and Practice* 2020 (April 1, 2020): 1–15. https://doi.org/10.1155/2020/5798285.

56. Shanahan, Catherine, and Luke Shanahan. *Deep Nutrition: Why Your Genes Need Traditional Food.* New York: Flatiron Books, 2017.

57. Dai, Danika, Courtney Miller, Violeta Valdivia, Brian Boyle, Paula Bolton, Shuang Li, Steve Seiner, and Robert Meisner. "Neurocognitive Effects of Repeated Ketamine Infusion Treatments in Patients with Treatment Resistant Depression: A Retrospective Chart Review." *BMC Psychiatry* 22, no. 1 (February 22, 2022): https://doi.org/10.1186/s12888-022-03789-3.

58. Can et al. "Low Dose Oral Ketamine Treatment."

59. Bolwig, Tom G., and Max Fink. "Electrotherapy for Melancholia." *Journal of ECT* 25, no. 1 (March 2009): 15–18. https://doi.org/10.1097/yct.0b013e318191b6e3.

60. Chesney, Edward, Guy M. Goodwin, and Seena Fazel. "Risks of All-Cause and Suicide Mortality in Mental Disorders: A Meta-Review." *World Psychiatry* 13, no. 2 (June 2014): 153–60. https://doi.org/10.1002/wps.20128.

61. Laursen, Thomas M., Trine Munk-Olsen, and Mogens Vestergaard. "Life Expectancy and Cardiovascular Mortality in Persons with Schizophrenia." *Current Opinion in Psychiatry* 25, no. 2 (March 2012): 83–88. https://doi.org/10.1097/yco.0b013e32835035ca.

CHAPTER 9

1. Sessa, Ben. "From Sacred Plants to Psychotherapy: The History and Re-Emergence of Psychedelics in Medicine." Paper presented at the Annual Meeting of the Royal College of Psychiatry's Spirituality in Psychiatry Special Interest Group, 2006.

Endnotes

https://www.rcpsych.ac.uk/docs/default-source/members/sigs/spirituality-spsig/ben-sessa-from-sacred-plants-to-psychotherapy.pdf?sfvrsn=d1bd0269_2.

2. Carhart-Harris, Robin L., and Guy M. Goodwin. "The Therapeutic Potential of Psychedelic Drugs: Past, Present, and Future." *Neuropsychopharmacology* 42, no. 11 (October 2017): 2105–13. https://doi.org/10.1038/npp.2017.84.

3. Pollan, Michael. *How to Change Your Mind: What the New Science of Psychedelics Teaches Us about Consciousness, Dying, Addiction, Depression, and Transcendence.* New York: Penguin Books, 2019.

4. Doblin, Richard E., Merete Christiansen, Lisa Jerome, and Brad Burge. "The Past and Future of Psychedelic Science: An Introduction to This Issue." *Journal of Psychoactive Drugs* 51, no. 2 (2019): 93–97. https://doi.org/10.1080/02791072.2019.1606472.

5. Peterson, Jordan B. *Beyond Order: 12 More Rules for Life.* New York: Penguin, 2022.

6. Kraehenmann, Rainer. "Dreams and Psychedelics: Neurophenomenological Comparison and Therapeutic Implications." *Current Neuropharmacology* 15, no. 7 (2017): 1032–42. https://doi.org/10.2174/1573413713666170619092629.

7. Nichols, David E. "Psychedelics." *Pharmacological Reviews* 68, no. 2 (April 2016): 264–355. https://doi.org/10.1124/pr.115.011478.

8. Carhart-Harris and Goodwin. "Therapeutic Potential of Psychedelic Drugs."

9. Doblin et al. "Past and Future of Psychedelic Science."

10. Barrett, Frederick S., and Roland R. Griffiths. "Classic Hallucinogens and Mystical Experiences: Phenomenology and Neural Correlates." In *Behavioral Neurobiology of Psychedelic Drugs* , eds. Adam Halberstadt, Franz X. Vollenweider, and David E. Nichols, 393–430. Vol. 36 of Current Topics in Behavioral Neurosciences. Cham, Switzerland: Springer, 2017. https://doi.org/10.1007/7854_2017_474.

11. Sanz, Camila, Federico Zamberlan, Earth Erowid, Fire Erowid, and Enzo Tagliazucchi. "The Experience Elicited by Hallucinogens Presents the Highest Similarity to Dreaming within a Large Database of Psychoactive Substance Reports." *Frontiers in Neuroscience* 12 (January 22, 2018): https://doi.org/10.3389/fnins.2018.00007.

12. Winkelman, Michael J. "The Mechanisms of Psychedelic Visionary Experiences: Hypotheses from Evolutionary Psychology." *Frontiers in Neuroscience* 11 (September 28, 2017): https://doi.org/10.3389/fnins.2017.00539.

13. Sanz et al. "Experience Elicited by Hallucinogens."

14. Wolfson, Phil. "Introduction." In *Ketamine Papers: Science, Therapy, and Transformation*, eds. Phil Wolfson and Glenn Hartelius, 293–94. Santa Cruz, CA: Multidisciplinary Association for Psychedelic Studies, 2016.

15. Friston, Karl. "The Free-Energy Principle: A Unified Brain Theory?" *Nature Reviews Neuroscience* 11, no. 2 (February 2010): 127–38. https://doi.org/10.1038/nrn2787.

16. van den Berg, Manon, Igor Magaraggia, Rudy Schreiber, Todd M. Hillhouse, and Joseph H. Porter. "How to Account for Hallucinations in the Interpretation of the Antidepressant Effects of Psychedelics: A Translational Framework." *Psychopharmacology* 239, no. 6 (June 2022): 1853–79. https://doi.org/10.1007/s00213-022-06106-8.

17. Erritzoe, David, James Smith, Patrick M. Fisher, Robin Carhart-Harris, Vibe G. Frokjaer, and Gitte M. Knudsen. "Recreational Use of Psychedelics Is Associated with Elevated Personality Trait Openness: Exploration of Associations with Brain Serotonin Markers." *Journal of Psychopharmacology* 33, no. 9 (2019): 1068–75. https://doi.org/10.1177/0269881119827891.

18. Knudsen, Gitte M. "Sustained Effects of Single Doses of Classical Psychedelics in Humans." *Neuropsychopharmacology* 48, no. 1 (January 2023): 145–50. https://doi.org/10.1038/s41386-022-01361-x.

19. Knudsen.

20. Mason, N. L., K. P. C. Kuypers, J. T. Reckweg, F. Müller, D. H. Y. Tse, B. Da Rios, S. W. Toennes, P. Stiers, A. Feilding, and J. G. Ramaekers. "Spontaneous and Deliberate Creative Cognition during and after Psilocybin Exposure." *Translational Psychiatry* 11 (April 8, 2021): https://doi.org/10.1038/s41398-021-01335-5.

21. Joules, R., O. M. Doyle, A. J. Schwarz, O. G. O'Daly, M. Brammer, S. C. Williams, and M. A. Mehta. "Ketamine Induces a Robust Whole-Brain Connectivity Pattern That Can Be Differentially Modulated by Drugs of Different Mechanism and Clinical Profile." *Psychopharmacology* 232, no. 21-22 (November 2015): 4205–18. https://doi.org/10.1007/s00213-015-3951-9.

22. Peterson. *Beyond Order.*

23. Mitchell, Jennifer M., Michael Bogenschutz, Alia Lilienstein, Charlotte Harrison, Sarah Kleiman, Kelly Parker-Guilbert, Marcela Ot'alora G., Wael Garas, Casey Paleos, Ingmar Gorman, Christopher Nicholas, Michael Mithoefer, Shannon Carlin, Bruce Poulter, Ann Mithoefer, Sylvestre Quevedo, Gregory Wells, Sukhpreet S. Klaire, Bessel van der Kolk, Keren Tzarfaty, Revital Amiaz, Ray Worthy, Scott Shannon, Joshua D. Woolley, Cole Marta, Yevgeniy Gelfand, Emma Hapke, Simon Amar, Yair Wallach, Randall Brown, Scott Hamilton, Julie B. Wang, Allison Coker, Rebecca Matthews, Alberdina de Boer, Berra Yazar-Klosinski, Amy Emerson, and Rick Doblin. "MDMA-Assisted Therapy for Severe PTSD: A Randomized, Double-Blind, Placebo-Controlled Phase 3 Study." *Nature Medicine* 27 (June 2021): 1025–33. https://doi.org/10.1038/s41591-021-01336-3.

24. Jansen, Karl. *Ketamine: Dreams and Realities.* Sarasota, FL: Multidisciplinary Association for Psychedelic Studies, 2004.

25. Sanz, Camila, Federico Zamberlan, Earth Erowid, Fire Erowid, and Enzo Tagliazucchi. "Corrigendum: The Experience Elicited by Hallucinogens Presents the Highest Similarity to Dreaming within a Large Database of Psychoactive Substance Reports." *Frontiers in Neuroscience* 12 (April 11, 2018): https://doi.org/10.3389/fnins.2018.00229.

26. Jansen. *Ketamine: Dreams and Realities.*

27. Sanz et al. "Corrigendum."

28. de Araujo, Draulio B., Sidarta Ribeiro, Guillermo A. Cecchi, Fabiana M. Carvalho, Tiago A. Sanchez, Joel P. Pinto, Bruno S. de Martinis, Jose A. Crippa, Jaime E. C. Hallak, and Antonio C. Santos. "Seeing with the Eyes Shut: Neural Basis of Enhanced Imagery Following Ayahuasca Ingestion." *Human Brain Mapping* 33, no. 11 (September 16, 2011): 2550–60. https://doi.org/10.1002/hbm.21381.

Endnotes

29. Wolfson, Phil. "Introduction."
30. Laven, David, dir. *Hamilton's Pharmacopeia*. Season 2, episode 5, "Ketamine; Realms and Realities." Aired December 26, 2017, on Viceland. https://www.vicetv.com/en_us/video/hamiltons-pharmacopeia-ketamine-realms-and-realities/59cd5d0b7752d1ac3e90aacf.
31. Hamilton, Jon. *Morning Edition*. "From Chaos to Calm: A Life Changed by Ketamine." National Public Radio, June 4, 2018, radio broadcast, audio, 6:24. https://www.npr.org/sections/health-shots/2018/06/04/615671405/from-chaos-to-calm-a-life-changed-by-ketamine.
32. Jansen. *Ketamine: Dreams and Realities*.
33. Jansen. *Ketamine: Dreams and Realities*. Kenneth Ring, author of *Life at Death*, classifies the near-death experience five-stage continuum.
34. Godoy, Daniel Agustin, Rafael Badenes, Paolo Pelosi, and Chiara Robba. "Ketamine in Acute Phase of Severe Traumatic Brain Injury 'an Old Drug for New Uses?'" *Critical Care* 25 (January 6, 2021): https://doi.org/10.1186/s13054-020-03452-x.
35. Feifel, David, David Dadiomov, and Kelly C. Lee. "Safety of Repeated Administration of Parenteral Ketamine for Depression." *Pharmaceuticals* 13, no. 7 (July 13, 2020): https://doi.org/10.3390/ph13070151.
36. Feifel, David, Benjamin Malcolm, Danielle Boggie, and Kelly Lee. "Low-Dose Ketamine for Treatment Resistant Depression in an Academic Clinical Practice Setting." *Journal of Affective Disorders* 221 (October 15, 2017): 283–88. https://doi.org/10.1016/j.jad.2017.06.043.
37. Green, S. M., K. J. Clem, and S. G. Rothrock. "Ketamine Safety Profile in the Developing World: Survey of Practitioners." *Academic Emergency Medicine* 3, no. 6 (June 1996): 598–604. https://pubmed.ncbi.nlm.nih.gov/8727631/.
38. Food and Drug Administration. "Ketalar (Ketamine Hydrochloride) Injection." Accessed January 9, 2023. https://www.accessdata.fda.gov/drugsatfda_docs/label/2017/016812s043lbl.pdf.
39. Strayer, Reuben J., and Lewis S. Nelson. "Adverse Events Associated with Ketamine for Procedural Sedation in Adults." *The American Journal of Emergency Medicine* 26, no. 9 (2008): 985–1028. https://doi.org/10.1016/j.ajem.2007.12.005.
40. Hyde, Stephen J. *Ketamine for Depression*. Self-published, Xlibris, 2015.
41. Feifel, Dadiomov, and Lee. "Safety of Repeated Administration."
42. McIntyre, Roger S., Joshua D. Rosenblat, Charles B. Nemeroff, Gerard Sanacora, James W. Murrough, Michael Berk, Elisa Brietzke, Seetal Dodd, Philip Gorwood, Roger Ho, Dan V. Iosifescu, Carlos Lopez Jaramillo, Siegfried Kasper, Kevin Kratiuk, Jung Goo Lee, Yena Lee, Leanna M. W. Lui, Rodrigo B. Mansur, George I. Papakostas, Mehala Subramaniapillai, Michael Thase, Eduard Vieta, Allan H. Young, Carlos Zarate Jr., and Stephen Stahl. "Synthesizing the Evidence for Ketamine and Esketamine in Treatment-Resistant Depression: An International Expert Opinion on the Available Evidence and Implementation." *American Journal of Psychiatry* 178, no. 5 (May 1, 2021): 383–99. https://doi.org/10.1176/appi. ajp.2020.20081251.

43. Edrich, Thomas, Andrew D. Friedrich, Holger K. Eltzschig, and Thomas W. Felbinger. "Ketamine for Long-Term Sedation and Analgesia of a Burn Patient." *Anesthesia & Analgesia* 99, no. 3 (September 2004): 893–95. https://doi.org/10.1213/01.ane.0000133002.42742.92.
44. Feifel et al. "Low-Dose Ketamine for Treatment Resistant Depression."
45. Edward F. Domino, and David S. Warner. "Taming the Ketamine Tiger." *Anesthesiology* 113, no. 3 (September 2010): 678–84. https://doi.org/10.1097/ALN.0b013e3181ed09a2.
46. Feifel et al. "Low-Dose Ketamine for Treatment Resistant Depression."
47. Walsh, Zach, Ozden Merve Mollaahmetoglu, Joseph Rootman, Shannon Golsof, Johanna Keeler, Beth Marsh, David J. Nutt, and Celia J. A. Morgan. "Ketamine for the Treatment of Mental Health and Substance Use Disorders: Comprehensive Systematic Review." *BJPsych Open* 8, no. 1 (2022): https://doi.org/10.1192/bjo.2021.1061.
48. Walsh, et al. "Ketamine for the Treatment of Mental Health and Substance Use Disorders."
49. Bylund, William, Liam Delahanty, and Maxwell Cooper. "The Case of Ketamine Allergy." *Clinical Practice and Cases in Emergency Medicine* 1, no. 4 (November 2017): 323–25. https://doi.org/10.5811/cpcem.2017.7.34405.
50. *Drugs and Lactation Database,* s.v. "Ketamine." National Library of Medicine, Last modified February 15, 2023. https://www.ncbi.nlm.nih.gov/books/NBK500566/.
51. Green, Clem, and Rothrock. "Ketamine Safety Profile."

CHAPTER 10

1. Hodges, Linda. "Why I Started a Ketamine Clinic." Medium.com, February 19, 2020. https://docmomtiredaf.medium.com/why-i-started-a-ketamine-clinic-4751b0b9b3a.
2. Feifel, David, Benjamin Malcolm, Danielle Boggie, and Kelly Lee. "Low-Dose Ketamine for Treatment Resistant Depression in an Academic Clinical Practice Setting." *Journal of Affective Disorders* 221 (October 15, 2017): 283–88. https://doi.org/10.1016/j.jad.2017.06.043.
3. "Mental Health Treatments in San Diego: TMS and Ketamine Therapy." Kadima Neuropsychiatry, n.d. https://www.kadimanp.com/.
4. Lieberman, Jeffrey A. "Back to the Future—the Therapeutic Potential of Psychedelic Drugs." *New England Journal of Medicine* 384 (April 15, 2021): 1460–61. https://doi.org/10.1056/nejme2102835.
5. Carhart-Harris, Robin, Bruna Giribaldi, Rosalind Watts, Michelle Baker-Jones, Ashleigh Murphy-Beiner, Roberta Murphy, Jonny Martell, Allan Blemings, David Erritzoe, and David J. Nutt. "Trial of Psilocybin versus Escitalopram for Depression." *New England Journal of Medicine* 384 (April 15, 2021): 1402–11. https://doi.org/10.1056/nejmoa2032994.

Index